The DASH Diet
Younger You

ALSO BY MARLA HELLER

The DASH Diet Action Plan

The DASH Diet Weight Loss Solution

The Everyday DASH Diet Cookbook

The DASH Diet Younger You

Shed 20 Years—and Pounds—
in Just 10 Weeks

Marla Heller, MS, RD

GRAND CENTRAL
Life & Style
NEW YORK · BOSTON

Grand Central Life & Style
Hachette Book Group
1290 Avenue of the Americas
New York, NY 10104

www.GrandCentralLifeandStyle.com

Printed in the United States of America

RRD-C

First Edition: December 2014
10 9 8 7 6 5 4 3 2 1

Grand Central Life & Style is an imprint of Grand Central Publishing. The Grand Central Life & Style name and logo are trademarks of Hachette Book Group, Inc.

The Hachette Speakers Bureau provides a wide range of authors for speaking events. To find out more, go to www.HachetteSpeakersBureau.com or call (866) 376-6591.

The publisher is not responsible for websites (or their content) that are not owned by the publisher.

Library of Congress Cataloging-in-Publication Data

Heller, Marla.
    The DASH diet younger you : shed 20 years—and pounds—in just 10 weeks / Marla Heller, MS, RD.—First edition.
        pages cm.
    Includes bibliographical references and index.
    ISBN 978-1-4555-5454-6 (hardcover)—ISBN 978-1-4789-8327-9 (audio download)—ISBN 978-1-4555-5453-9 (ebook) 1. Reducing diets—Recipes. 2. Aging—Prevention—Nutritional aspects. 3. Aging—Diet therapy—Recipes. I. Title.
    RM222.2.H361813 2015
    613.2'5—dc23
                                                                                          2014020883

            ISBN 978-1-4789-8686-7 (audiobook)

To my loving, inspiring, and, oh-so-patient husband,
Richard Heller

CONTENTS

PART III
Breakthrough Lifestyle Solutions

INTRODUCTION

Tick, tock. Tick, tock.

That's the sound of time ticking by, and with it your internal clock, the one that determines your chronological age. Many people fear the ticking of that clock, thinking it will bring with it the frustrating effects of aging, like joint pain, weight gain (especially that stubborn belly weight!), wrinkles, and age-related illnesses.

But you don't have to be at the mercy of the clock! Those age-related consequences are avoidable! You can choose to stop the march of time that defines chronological aging and hold firm instead—and indefinitely—to the inner and outer youthfulness we naturally enjoy in our younger years. Whether you're in your twenties or thirties and are focused on keeping your youthful energy, health, and looks, or you're in your forties, fifties, or older and want to reverse the signs of aging and recover that inward and outward resilience you enjoyed in your younger years, *The DASH Diet Younger You* puts you back in the driver's seat. Your youthfulness no longer has to have an expiration date!

That's because this plan stems from the most trusted and effective program in diets: the DASH diet. The DASH (Dietary Approaches to Stop Hypertension) diet has been named the Best Overall Diet and the Healthiest Diet by *U.S. News & World Report*.

The health benefits of DASH are well documented and well known. It lowers blood pressure in fourteen days. It lowers cholesterol and preserves brain function. It lowers the rates of heart attack, stroke, heart failure, and some types of cancer, including BRCA-negative breast cancer. And if you follow the DASH program, you're less likely to develop diabetes or kidney stones.

And now, thanks to exciting new research, I have discovered how the DASH Diet can be your anti-aging solution, too! This plan is specifically designed to help you shed not just pounds but also years, with a program of renewal and rejuvenation that will deliver a *younger* you—in as little as ten weeks.

The desire for eternal youth—an enduring wish to continue to look and feel young—is as old as time itself. The quest to find the secrets of everlasting youth and beauty stretches as far back as recorded history; most notably, it inspired the Spanish explorer Ponce de León to comb the world for a fountain of youth. The road to this promised land has been littered by fairy tales and false leads. The fountain of youth, though, is not to be found in some mystical, far-flung land; the secrets to maintaining our youthfulness can be found in the same fertile bedrock of science and nutrition that drives our medical frontiers forward. In fact, exciting research from the past few years reveals the tools you need to understand and control the mechanisms of aging—all through changes in diet and lifestyle.

Drawing on this research, in conjunction with my own decades of experience as an expert and pioneer in bringing the DASH diet to the public, I've created a brand-new DASH anti-aging program: *The DASH Diet Younger You* plan. With this book as your guide, you'll learn the latest secrets to looking and feeling younger and reversing the signs of premature aging—secrets that are simpler than you may think.

You've picked up this book because you, too, are interested in stopping or turning back the clock. Great news: This program will get you to that goal—in as little as ten weeks.

Let me tell you how and why. I'm a registered dietitian with twenty years of experience working hands-on with thousands of clients. Combined with my many years of postgraduate education, I've developed expertise in nutrition and the prevention of disease, and I had the privilege of working with one of the original architects of the DASH diet. I was tasked with creating a program to implement DASH for the public—in other words, to make the first scientifically proven diet easy to use for busy people in the real world. I was happy to share the DASH program with readers nationwide in my *New York Times* bestselling books, *The DASH Diet Action Plan, The DASH Diet Weight Loss Solution*, and *The Everyday DASH Diet Cookbook*. Crowned the #1 diet by *U.S. News & World Report* for several years running, DASH came to fame as the diet proven to be as effective as front-line medications in preventing or reversing hypertension, diabetes, heart disease, and even some cancers. Were it not for the endorsements of the National Institutes of Health (NIH), the American Heart Association, and the Mayo Clinic, along with a legion of doctors, such claims might be dismissed as nothing more than the hyperbole we have come to expect from passing diet fads. But the DASH diet is for real.

For me, the most important thing about DASH is that it proves that dietary intervention alone can have the same (or greater!) efficacy as prescription medications in fighting disease, minus all the nasty side effects and costly price tag! Since DASH has the ability to fight back diseases like hypertension and diabetes, I knew those same mechanisms held the promise—if harnessed correctly—of even more benefits. The same health-restoring properties in DASH that allow us to stave off disease can be amped up to go that achievement one better, and actually hold back the conditions we associate with aging.

That is what inspired me to create this amazing, easy, and effective anti-aging program. In my first books, I brought the benefits of the original DASH to the public and made it so easy to follow. But I have long realized that the DASH diet has so much more potential, not just to make us healthier and slimmer, but also to make us younger! To design this new program, I went back to the foundational research and reexamined every DASH study to discover how to maximize the benefits and rev up those properties necessary to keep us youthful and to restore us to our prime—inside and out!—indefinitely.

In creating this program, I incorporated remarkable benefits mined from newer research on how to preserve youthfulness and health—studies that were not available when DASH was originally developed. I discovered that the right foods, in the right proportions, can actually slow the processes of aging, even postpone and reverse them. How? By stopping damage at the cellular and DNA level before it causes wrinkles, sagging skin, excess fat around the waist, memory loss, and other symptoms traditionally associated with aging. These and other conditions, once thought to be the inevitable baggage we will carry as we advance in years, can actually be delayed or halted. Once I identified which foods had the greatest benefits, I knew I was onto something groundbreaking. I kept the foundation of the DASH diet as a basis for what I knew could be a revolutionary approach to anti-aging. After all, DASH has a research and medical pedigree like no other diet, along with the chops to halt disease in its tracks. To understand from the inside how a "mere" food intervention can reverse and prevent disease is to see the potential for turning back not only the diseases of aging, but aging itself.

This new research is mind-blowing. Case in point: Researchers are studying pieces of DNA called telomeres, which are directly involved in the aging process, both as markers and as influencers of aging. The longer your telomeres, the more youthful you will stay and the better you'll be able to sidestep the diseases of aging. The strategies you'll implement in this program will actually preserve the length of your telomeres—and this all leads to a younger you.

Scientists have also discovered that a healthy gut with the right balance of friendly bacteria carries benefits far beyond good digestion. These "good bugs" also make it easier to reach and maintain a healthy weight, improve mood, boost immunity, and even repair sun-damaged skin! And a healthy gut fully absorbs trace micronutrients that are important for youth, vitality, and health. The DASH Diet Younger You plan is brimming with foods that will make you more youthful from the inside out.

In the 1990s, stale advice harped that "all foods can fit" and recommended that sugar, along with processed foods, could be part of a healthy diet. Well, that tired advice led to the epidemics of diabetes and obesity we are struggling with today. Not only are these major health problems, but we are also finding that sugar can disrupt hunger hormones and cause inflammation, which increases your odds of heart disease, dementia, and other illnesses associated with aging.

Let's never forget: Youthfulness is associated with less disease. There is a physiological correlation between aging and disease. While young, most people are not plagued by chronic disease. On the other hand, if you're dealing with diseases such as high blood pressure, cardiovascular disease, or diabetes, it is an indication that your body is actually aging faster than it needs to. What's worse is that if you are taking medications to treat any of these diseases, the side effects of those meds can actually accelerate aging.

But don't worry: I'll show you how diet and lifestyle changes can help restore a healthy baseline, so that you may be able to get off those drugs, or at least cut back on your dosages (always and only after consulting with your doctor, of course!). Take blood pressure, for example. The original DASH diet is widely prescribed for hypertension. In fact, it is proven to lower blood pressure in fourteen days, and that's without medication. And therein lies one of DASH's amazing secrets: Biologically, as opposed to chronologically, people with healthy blood pressure are up to twenty-five years younger than people with high blood pressure. In other words, if you and your best friend are both forty-five and you have high blood pressure and hers is normal, your body is more like the body of someone who is seventy years old. Your friend's body seems twenty-five years younger! Just by eating the right foods in the right ratios and making some specific, but simple, changes to your lifestyle, you can turn back the clock, too!

How fabulous, then, to have a diet and lifestyle plan that is prescription strength but doesn't have any negative side effects! Instead, it has spectacular collateral benefits. This new and improved DASH program can inoculate you against aging—and prevent the diseases of aging.

In this book, I introduce five groundbreaking, age-defying strategies, and I show you how to start implementing them right away, starting today.

The first strategy is that on this new plan, you'll eat more plant-based meals than you might have in the past. A plant-based diet positively affects every organ in your body, from your skin to your heart to your brain. This means a longer life, and just as important, it means turning back the clock, so that you'll be enjoying those "extra" years with youthful vitality, inside and out.

My goal in the DASH Diet Younger You plan is to provide you with a program that can deliver all the advantages of a plant-focused diet while still being flexible enough to also appeal to the majority of Americans, who do not wish to give up meat completely.

Second, you'll harness the power of anti-aging compounds in foods called flavonoids. The science behind the anti-aging capacity of flavonoids has only recently been uncovered. These plant powerhouse chemicals affect your body at the DNA level to keep you youthful.

Third, you'll naturally detox by emphasizing foods that promote the friendly bacteria that restore your system to a healthy, younger state.

Fourth, you'll learn to avoid the refined starches and sugars that have recently been found to be aging stimulators.

Fifth, you'll get off processed foods that can speed up aging and find a delicious, clean way of eating. Along with this fifth strategy, you'll become healthier and less dependent on certain age-promoting drugs, and you may be able to get off them altogether. The DASH food pattern—including every nutrient, every microcomponent, and each type of food on this diet, working in sync—confers youth-giving benefits.

I introduced the new plan to my practice, and the results were amazing. Clients who followed it *for just one month* reported that they were flooded with compliments about their appearance, from remarks that they looked younger to raves about glowing skin, shiny hair, and clear eyes. "Have you been to a spa?" friends asked, or in more hushed tones, "Did you have work done?" In addition to shedding years, my clients also shed excess pounds, bringing them back to a rejuvenated, more youthful appearance. Still others were sharper in their thinking and stronger in their bodies, with more youthful posture. I watched people get younger right before my eyes, as if the process of aging had not only stopped, but seemed to be going in reverse.

There's more to this program than just the diet. There's a life-style component that urges you to make some changes in the way you live. But I'm not offering up the same tired advice you've heard a million times. No. I'll show you how certain activities directly affect your DNA, reverse the primary processes of aging, and in effect, stop you from aging. This is information that has been only recently discovered by science—and it works synergistically with the diet. I will also help you "own" the DASH Diet Younger You program, whether you are concerned about sidestepping wrinkles, defying "old age" illnesses, or everything in between. And because the plan is based on foods and lifestyle, you don't have to wait for a drug company to develop a new product—you can take advantage of this program today!

My plan is proven to help reverse the inward and outward signs of aging. In less than one month you will start to see and feel the difference. In only two months, you will truly be younger and healthier.

Your payoffs will be immense: a youthful appearance that will have you turning heads; strength; vitality; and, ultimately, a healthier and more vibrant life. While you're enjoying your new way of eating and its amazing rewards, I'll talk to you about all the anti-aging benefits you can expect to enjoy, such as:

- Healthier, younger-looking hair, skin, and nails
- Clearer, healthier eyes
- Weight loss, especially around your tummy
- A healthier heart and blood pressure
- A more nimble brain that defies dementia
- A higher libido and a sexier body
- Protection against diabetes and even some kinds of cancer
- Stronger bones and muscles and more flexible joints

You'll also learn how to make the DASH Diet Younger You program a way of life for you and your family.

I often envision a world where men and women of all ages can recover their energy and health to live at their peak, indefinitely. In other words, I imagine a world where we remain wrinkle free and gloriously youthful despite the march of time. I know it sounds impossible, like a fantasy. But maybe not. In fact, researchers have taken giant steps toward unveiling the secrets underlying the aging process and toward preventing its changes through proven anti-aging strategies—paving the way for longer, healthier lives!

The DASH Diet Younger You plan can help you get there. This book brings you the good news that science and nutrition have delivered us to the promised land of longer life and enduring youthfulness, inside and out. This happily-ever-after is no longer simply the stuff of fairy tales or hucksters' spiels. Chronological age can be deceiving. I know plenty of people in their thirties and forties who look (and feel) decades older. I also see lots of people in their sixties or seventies who look (and live) decades younger. The prematurely old have accelerated their aging process because they've succumbed to the poor nutritional and lifestyle choices of our times. But I also know that when they decide to change their diets and their lives, they can reclaim their youthfulness—they will no longer look older than their years, but, perhaps, much younger.

You can join the ranks of the new order of eternal "youngsters" with the right diet and the right plan, and that plan is the DASH Diet Younger You.

Are you ready to start getting younger?

—*Marla Heller*

The DASH Diet
Younger You

PART I

DASH to a Younger You

CHAPTER 1

You Are As Young As You Eat

Think of your body as a symphony orchestra, with all your cells, tissues, and organs as instruments. The music they play comprises you and everything you do. When your "instruments" are playing in harmony, you look and feel young. But as you get older, your music starts to drift off-key. Over time, the music gets out of tune. Then you start aging.

You know the signs of an off-key body: wrinkles, sagging skin, a poochy belly, sagging shoulders, and thinning, gray hair. These signs are visible; others are not so visible. They're occurring inside your body, right down to the cellular level. Your blood pressure may rise as you get older. Your body can't process sugar as well. You gradually lose muscle and bone, while packing on body fat. Your shape changes, with that fat filling in where muscle used to be. Medical exams might show that your heart isn't pumping as well as it used to, your kidneys may not be working as efficiently, and your lung power has fallen off. And then there is one of the most critical manifestations of human aging—the decline of your immune system.

All of this, inside and out, strikes an alarming chord. So what's going on? What causes aging?

For centuries, aging has been thought to be an inescapable breakdown of the body and its organs. Much like a car with too many miles on it, the human machine eventually wears out. You can keep repairing the parts and getting tune-ups, but eventually the vehicle stops running.

There's nothing much you can do about it. Or is there?

I'm absolutely convinced we can extend human life—and the quality of that life. This is not science fiction. Although the anti-aging science behind this plan is just newly discovered, which has allowed me to optimize my plan, the foundation of the DASH Diet Younger You plan is one that I have perfected with the thousands of people I have worked with over my twenty-year career. So I have seen the results and know that there's a lot you can do to slow down, postpone, even reverse aging. We know so much more about what causes aging than ever before. But the best news of all is that with measures as simple as diet, exercise, and lifestyle changes, we can stop three key processes that cause aging.

What are those key processes? Let's take a look.

Oxid-Aging

One of the most prevalent and credible theories of aging is that our cells are increasingly damaged, the older we get, by what are called free radicals. Free radicals are renegade molecules created by the normal process of burning food and oxygen to make energy. Unchecked, they assault the body through oxidative damage, or oxidation, a process that literally rusts us from the inside out. Free radicals can wrinkle your skin and harm your heart. At a more fundamental level, these errant molecules chip away at the DNA in cells, possibly mutating the genetic code, which can increase the risk of developing cancer. Once this DNA wreckage occurs, it's likely to be permanent and will accelerate the aging process. This is what "oxid-aging" is all about.

Fortunately, cells can fight back with antioxidants that detoxify free radicals. The most famous antioxidants are vitamins C and E, but there are many more nutrients in plant foods that also act as natural, powerful antioxidants, from minerals to phytochemicals (natural substances in plants that fight disease). The body also has its own cavalry of natural antioxidants. In fact, the reason humans live longer than most species is because we have unusually high levels of antioxidants in our bodies. Even so, it is up to us to help our antioxidant defenses stay strong through diet and exercise. Unless we do, free radicals will outnumber antioxidants, and that's what creates oxid-aging.

We can prevent oxid-aging by eating foods plentiful in antioxidants. Vitamin E from nuts and seeds, and beta-carotene from orange and yellow vegetables, trap and neutralize free radicals physically, by lying in wait in the membranes that surround the cell nucleus. They go to work against cholesterol, too. You can't see it or taste it, but cholesterol is in all foods of animal origin, foods like eggs, poultry, meat, and fish, and it is produced in your body utilizing fats from animal sources and from plant foods. One reason cholesterol leads to heart disease is that it becomes oxidized by free radicals in the arteries. Antioxidants, including vitamin C and many phytochemicals, help prevent oxidation of cholesterol.

The foods you'll be eating on the DASH Diet Younger You program are loaded with antioxidants that stay on the lookout for free radicals and squelch them before they can do damage.

Physical activity also helps. At first, exercise can stimulate free radicals, but as your muscles adapt to regular activity and grow stronger, they increase the production of natural antioxidants.

You can thus stop oxid-aging easily—and in doing so, improve your health and increase your longevity.

Inflamm-Aging

"Inflamm-aging" is a term coined by scientists to describe how chronic inflammation affects aging. When something injures or infects our body, immune cells are pressed into service immediately. Like cellular EMTs (Emergency Medical Technicians), they rush through the bloodstream to the injury site or to confront invading germs. You can see this rescue process in action when an injured area feels warm or looks red and swollen. This reaction is referred to as acute inflammation. It's a perfectly normal response, designed to heal the body. Acute inflammation can last from hours to days. As it subsides, the rescuer cells perish or are disbanded. You are healed and back to normal.

But if this immune response continues, the body goes into a state of ongoing inflammation. This is called chronic inflammation, and it underlies most serious diseases.

Arthritis is one disease related to inflammation. So are heart disease, dementia, and type 2 diabetes. Even excess weight can be part of the inflammation response, both by aggravating it and by serving as a response to inflammation.

When scientists talk about inflamm-aging, they're referring to the shortening of telomeres, which is caused by inflammation. Telomeres are caps that protect the ends of your chromosomes, in much the same way as the plastic tips of your shoelaces keep them from fraying. When the telomeres shorten too much, the cell stops dividing and dies off (a process termed apoptosis). Undersized telomeres are associated with heart disease, cancer, dementia, and early death.

Numerous studies suggest that a plant-focused diet like the DASH Diet Younger You plan, full of foods like vegetables, fruits, and beans, can decrease inflammation and thus protect telomeres and prevent them from shortening.

Beware Hormone Hype

What about hormones? Do they affect the aging process? Yes, the levels of certain hormones do drop off as we get older. A lot of so-called anti-aging clinics promote taking hormones to "cure" aging. Among the hormones they push are human growth hormone (HGH) and dehydroepiandrosterone (DHEA)—two substances that our bodies produce less of as we age. The theory is, if these hormones were at their height in our young bodies, why not take hormone supplements as time marches on? In fact, there have been some reports of gains in endurance and muscle, and reduced body fat, from taking these drugs. But people who took them had also had an increase in certain problems, including arthritis and diabetes—two diseases of aging. Estrogen and progesterone replacement is controversial, too, and may lead to heart disease and increased risk for stroke— additional diseases of aging. The DASH Diet Younger You plan is about turning back the clock using food and lifestyle, not drugs or supplemental hormones.

Glyc-Aging

The third aging process is called glycation, or more aptly, glyc-aging. As we get older, we don't process sugar as well. We may develop prediabetes symptoms, even if we don't have the full-blown disease. Excess sugar molecules amass in the blood, tying up with proteins such as collagen in the skin, or proteins in the brain. This process produces advanced glycation end products (AGEs), which cause wrinkles, promote inflammation (which hurts immunity), and accelerate aging. AGEs can also make you prone to developing diabetes, heart disease, dementia, and other diseases of aging. In my work with people with diabetes, I always noticed accelerated aging in those whose sugar levels were not under control. And, of course, you don't have to be diabetic for sugars to speed aging in your body.

To understand glycation, think of what happens when you grill a steak. After the proteins in the meat are exposed to high heat, the meat gets crusty or crispy because naturally occurring sugars caramelize and bind to the protein molecules.

The very same thing happens to our skin and organs once sugar enters the bloodstream and links itself to collagen in a process called cross-linking. Collagen is an important protein that holds together cells, tissues, and organs and is a major constituent of your skin, bone, cartilage, and tendons. With cross-linking, AGEs cause collagen molecules to stick together. As a result, once-healthy collagen fibers lose their elasticity, becoming rigid, stiff, and brittle. The effect is most apparent in wrinkled skin, a cardinal sign of growing older. Even if you're healthy, the effects of glycation on your skin can show up when you're around thirty-five and get progressively worse after that, according to a 2001 study in the *British Journal of Dermatology*. Glycation can also hurt organs whose flexibility is important, such as the heart, kidneys, brain, skin, and eyes.

AGEs can occur in foods, especially in fried and cooked meats, and they are associated with increased risk for dementia and diabetes. AGEs promote the accumulation of amyloid plaques—sprawling tangles of protein molecules in the brain—that are characteristic of Alzheimer's disease.

When we're younger, our immune system cells act as garbage collectors, removing sugar-linked proteins; but with the passage of time, the cells cannot keep up. And as soon as sugar causes proteins to cross-link, glyc-aging begins.

The DASH Diet Younger You plan combats this cycle of

damage. It helps you avoid foods with added sugars and high-fat meats, keeps your blood sugar under control, and adds foods high in nutrients known to prevent glyc-aging.

DASH Wrinkles

One of the best, but toughest, ways to stop wrinkles is to quit smoking. Each puff you take contains billions and billions of free radicals. Nicotine suffocates the skin, causing it to deteriorate. Cigarettes contain thousands of chemicals that destroy elastin and collagen, the proteins that make your skin taut and wrinkle free. The act of smoking—with its puckering and blowing—also creates "dynamic" wrinkles, those caused by repetitive motion. Smoking also shortens telomeres. Quit smoking to prevent further damage, and allow the DASH diet's good nutrition to start repairing your skin.

Eat Your Way to Youth

All three of these aging processes are affected by and can be reversed by the five nutritional strategies that form the heart of my DASH anti-aging program:

1. **Eat a plant-focused diet.** The DASH Diet Younger You plan is rich in fruits and vegetables, whole grains, beans, nuts, and seeds. Of course, you do get to eat other healthy foods, such as low-fat and nonfat dairy foods, heart-healthy fats, and the healthiest protein-rich foods, which can include fish, poultry, and eggs. Or you can choose to go totally vegetarian if you prefer. Plant foods are the centerpiece because, as you'll learn, they combat all three processes of aging.

The scientific proof is remarkable: People who follow a plant-focused style of eating live longer; people who eat more vegetables and fruits tend to have fewer wrinkles and more attractive skin; and plant-based diets offer protection from diseases of aging such as cancer and heart disease.

2. **Focus on flavonoids.** One reason plant foods are so powerful against aging is that they are chock-full of powerful chemicals that protect you. Among these chemicals are flavonoids, which give fruits and vegetables their color. Flavonoids work as antioxidants to fight free radicals, and they have recently been found to help lengthen telomeres.

3. **Populate your diet with probiotics and prebiotics.** These substances help maintain a healthy, stable "microbiota" in your system—the normal ratio of good bacteria to bad—to keep your all-important digestive system working to the max. You'll do that by adding fermented foods like yogurt and fibrous foods like beans, nuts, fruits, and vegetables to your diet.

4. **Avoid damaging sugars.** Refined sugar is everywhere in processed foods, and it really is making us old before our time, inside and out. The DASH Diet Younger You plan will help you get off sugar so you can get on with healthy, youthful living.

5. **Fire Big Food and Big Pharma.** The processed foods you've been eating, and some of the drugs you've been prescribed, are aging you. The foods most people eat today are products of the huge food industry, often called Big Food, which churns out food made with synthetic chemicals, additives, extra sugars, refined grains, fats, and more—all of which make us sick and old. Soda has replaced milk on the family dinner table. Meat now comes mostly from livestock that has been fattened with hormones and antibiotics. "Fake"

foods that are low-fat or low-sugar have duped us into eating even more processed foods because they sound healthy but in fact are far less satisfying. Not to mention that these foods contain a host of chemicals and additives that keep the food shelf-stable but aren't that healthy for us to consume.

The same is true of the ginormous pharmaceutical industry. Many of the drugs we're prescribed on a regular basis are designed to treat lifestyle diseases, but in many cases healthy food and exercise can work just as well as, if not better than, these medicines. Many of the medications used to treat these diseases make you older-appearing and older-feeling. Even worse, some of those meds can actually increase your risk for developing the other diseases of aging.

The DASH Diet Younger You plan is a return to basic, real foods eating. Once you've stepped out of the world of overprocessed foods, you'll see how easy it is to reclaim your youth.

Is Your Present Diet Aging You? Take This 5-Point Quiz

This is a multiple-choice quiz. Read through each question, circling the letter that best fits your response. Answer as accurately as possible.

1. During a typical week, how often do you eat potato chips, corn chips, crackers, or similar snack foods, or French fries?
   A. Rarely
   B. Once
   C. More than twice

(continued)

2. During a typical week, how often do you eat doughnuts, sugary pastries, or desserts?
   A. Rarely
   B. Once
   C. More than twice

3. During a typical week, how often do you eat processed meats such as hot dogs, bacon, pepperoni, luncheon meats—or even the reduced-fat versions of these foods?
   A. Rarely
   B. Once
   C. More than twice

4. During a typical week, how much fatty meat do you eat? (Examples of fatty meat include rib-eye, T-bone, and porterhouse steaks; hamburgers; and even most turkey burgers.)
   A. Rarely
   B. Once
   C. More than twice

5. During a typical week, how many alcoholic beverages do you consume?
   A. Rarely do I consume alcoholic beverages.
   B. One drink a day but no less
   C. More than one drink daily

Scoring:

For every A you answered, give yourself 3 points.
For every B you answered, give yourself 1 point.
For every C you answered, give yourself 0 points.

Analysis:

Score of 12 to 15: Congratulations! You are younger than your years, and you probably look young, too. Keep up the good work: Avoid processed foods and fatty meats, stay off sugar, and keep your alcohol intake low. This book will teach you additional techniques to turn back the clock and maintain your youthfulness and vitality.

Score of 8 to 11: You're doing a great job to preserve your youth. To do even better, examine areas in which you may be faltering—too many processed foods, too much fat, or too much alcohol in your weekly diet—and cut back accordingly. This book will provide you with a comprehensive plan to do so!

Score of 0 to 7: You may be starting to feel the signs of unhealthy lifestyle choices or see them in the mirror, but no need to worry: This book is here to help! Start eating more fresh and unprocessed foods, reduce saturated and trans fats, and cut back on alcohol consumption. Get on the DASH Diet Younger You plan right away. Follow its principles and expect to be a younger you in no time.

The DASH Diet Younger You Plan: What to Expect

Allow me to share with you the benefits and changes I have seen in many people whom I have put on this plan. Expect the same wonderful changes to happen to you.

Natural Weight Loss

You may have seen it in others or experienced it yourself—the scale slowly inches up and up as the years go by. For too many people, the pounds seem to pile on as they get older. Aging slows metabolism, so weight gain is definitely a sign of getting older.

Excess weight in turn ages us in so many ways. It strains our joints and aggravates back problems. It leads to fatty liver and gallbladder problems. It makes us more likely to have sleep apnea. It increases our risks for several types of cancer, diabetes, heart disease, and strokes. All of these problems contribute to an older body.

But you don't have to put on pounds with age. In fact, you can look—and feel—even better than you did in your twenties by following this plan!

For one thing, the plant foods you'll be eating are naturally more satisfying, with fewer calories than foods in the standard American diet. That's because they're high in water and fiber, so that you feel full longer. The fiber in beans, for example, soaks up and helps escort fat and calories from your system. Heart-healthy fats found in foods like avocados, nuts, and seeds slow digestion, so that you're getting energy from your meals longer, and help to quench hunger pangs. This combination of food helps you avoid overeating, naturally.

Further, the calories on this plan are relatively low for the quantity of food you get to eat, which will help you reverse the weight gain that often comes with aging. But you don't have to focus on food labels or count calories or carb grams. You don't have to go to the grocery store with a calculator and a magnifying glass. All you have to do is eat the plant-based foods emphasized on the diet, with its foundation in vegetables and fruits, along with nuts, beans, and seeds.

By ditching processed foods, refined grains, and foods with added sugars, you'll naturally get rid of the constellation of metabolic changes that cause belly fat and have forced your body to become a fat-storing machine.

I DASHed Aging!

I've been overweight most of my adult life. At age forty-four, I was looking old and dowdy—and feeling desperate. Although I've been on a million diets, I decided to try the DASH Diet Younger You plan.

I started it, promising myself that I wouldn't get on the scale for seven days. But I wanted to see if this plan was really working. So on day two, I hopped on the scale. I had lost three pounds! I couldn't believe it. I actually cried, since this was the first time I had ever seen the scale go down.

My goal is to not have to go to the big-girl stores to buy my jeans anymore. I want to buy and wear a pair of skinny jeans and walk around in them, feeling confident and beautiful.

—*Ellen T.*

Youthful Beauty

The DASH Diet Younger You plan is rich in nutrients that beautify skin, hair, and nails, and you'll see the benefits of eating these foods very quickly after starting the program. Too many Americans eat diets that are deficient in the key vitamins and minerals that protect our outer beauty. Admittedly, I've been the victim of these deficiencies. My own physician noticed my breaking nails and realized that I was probably deficient in vitamin D, which my lab tests confirmed. After I started emphasizing foods rich in vitamin D, my nails became stronger and stopped splitting.

A diet rich in fruits and vegetables naturally improves skin tone while zapping the aging effects of oxidants in our environment. Getting sufficient protein is also key to preserving skin, hair, and nail health. With this plan, you get the complete package for looking and feeling younger.

DASH to the Bedroom: Rejuvenate Your Sex Life

In recent years, several studies have looked into the role of diet on erectile dysfunction (ED) and libido. Basically, what they've found is that a diet high in fruits, vegetables, and other plant foods, but low in red and processed meats and refined starches and sugar, helps resolve ED and boost libido. You'll find those dietary choices in the DASH Diet Younger You plan.

Such discoveries don't surprise me. The blood-pressure- and cholesterol-lowering benefits of the DASH plan mean that there will be greater blood flow in your whole body, including to your nether regions. That goes for both men and women. With more blood flow, there is more lubrication, greater arousal, and more powerful orgasms.

Plus, you'll just have more energy for everything—including sex—when you ditch the fatty junk food. So help yourself to a second and third serving of veggies. Your sex drive will love it—and your partner will, too.

Young at Heart and in Body

The DASH Diet Younger You plan guards against hypertension, stroke, heart problems, diabetes, and cancer—chronic diseases that tend to strike us later in life.

The heart of the DASH program is its blood-pressure-lowering benefit. As I mentioned, DASH stands for Dietary Approaches to Stop Hypertension. It was developed to be the healthiest American diet, offering all the heart-healthy benefits of a vegetarian diet, but still flexible enough to appeal to everyone. And that it does.

Research has shown that DASH can abolish nearly thirty years of "blood pressure aging" in just two weeks! High blood pressure is aging, as are the medications used to treat it. The DASH diet is the only diet proven in research to lower blood pressure so fast. It is so powerful that it is recommended for all patients who are newly diagnosed with high blood pressure.

Lower blood pressure is associated with more flexible veins and arteries, which helps keep your body younger from the inside out. Healthy, unclogged blood vessels are better able to bring nourishment to your entire body, including skin, eyes, and sex organs.

Long-term studies of thousands of people have proved beyond a shadow of a doubt that DASH lowers rates of heart attacks, strokes, and heart failure. People who follow a DASH-style eating pattern have a dramatically lower risk of developing type 2 diabetes. And the DASH eating pattern is tied to a lower risk of several types of cancer, including BRCA-negative breast cancer (this is a cancer with no familial link).

I DASHed Aging!

I'm fifty-two. In three months on this plan, I lost twenty-three pounds, scaled down five points off my body fat percentage, and trimmed 4.5 inches from my waist—all after struggling with my weight for decades.

At my physical today, my doctor looked at my blood work and said, "Wait, how old are you?! These are some of the best blood numbers I've seen all month in anyone." My overall cholesterol was 121, down from 160+; my triglycerides were 106; and my LDL was 64. He said I had the numbers of a healthy twenty-year-old. And that's exactly how I feel!

—Serena J.

Brain Youth

You may think of age-related memory and mental declines as inevitable, but I bring good news: The DASH diet has been shown in scientific studies to preserve memory and to be associated with lower risk of dementia as we get older. One primary reason is that DASH helps keep blood pressure in a healthy range. This, in turn, helps keep arteries clean, thus promoting good blood flow to the brain. Add in lots of plant antioxidants and skip added sugars to preserve healthy brain tissue with this plan, and the net effect is a younger brain.

Bone Strength

Few conditions are more aging than having to hunch over from spinal compression fractures or becoming immobilized after a hip fracture—both signs of aging bones. On the DASH Diet Younger You plan, you'll be taking in plenty of calcium and vitamin D for bone protection. What's more, you'll be consuming other bone-protective nutrients, such as protein and magnesium from dairy foods. Add more physical activity, and you will rejuvenate your bones. If you were lucky, your mother used to tell you to drink your milk. I am going to reaffirm that advice.

I hope I've given you powerful motivation to get started—and to start getting younger. It's never too late. With this plan, you'll add not just more years to your life, but also more life to your years.

CHAPTER 2

Pump Up Plant-Based Eating

The fountain of youth is no longer a legendary place or a magical elixir. It's a diet-centered approach to health that focuses on longevity-promoting foods, especially fruits and vegetables. Listen, you already know these foods are good for you. You heard it from your mother first: Eat your fruits and vegetables! But for those of you who got to the party late, these foods are miracle workers. They aren't fattening, and they provide the vitamins, minerals, and other nutrients you need for life. But now there's an even better reason to eat your fruits and veggies: They will keep you young. No kidding!

People who follow a plant-focused style of eating will tend to:

- Live longer.
- Have fewer wrinkles and more attractive skin.
- Be protected from chronic life-shortening diseases, such as heart disease, arthritis, Alzheimer's, and other diseases of aging.

- Have no trouble controlling their weight and staying in great shape. That's important, because a slimmer you is a younger you.

The discoveries being made about the anti-aging benefits of plant foods are nothing short of miraculous. They turn back the clock in two main ways—by fighting inflamm-aging and oxid-aging.

Plants Fight Inflamm-Aging

Years ago, while I was researching DASH and anti-aging, I thought that once you started getting older, it could only get worse, that "anti-aging" was more hype than hope. I was wrong. You can stop this process, easily.

How?

By pumping up the plant foods in your diet—which is exactly what the DASH Diet Younger You plan does. In breakthrough research, investigators have shown that when you switch to a plant-based diet, your body resists inflamm-aging.

As I pointed out in the previous chapter, chronic inflammation shortens telomeres, the segments of DNA that protectively cap the ends of chromosomes. Each time a cell undergoes division, a small piece of telomere is snipped off in the process. When telomeres get too short, cells stop replicating, start to malfunction, and eventually die. Think of this as being like a printer slowly running out of ink. Each new page becomes fainter, and less true to what it should be. The same is true for cell replication. As more and more cells die, the results include wrinkling and the general decline that is aging.

Eating more fruits and vegetables performs two amazing anti-aging feats: It helps lengthen telomeres and it helps create more telomerase, an enzyme that rebuilds telomeres and prevents chromosomes from degrading. You actually get younger at the cellular level.

In a study involving thirty-five men in their fifties and sixties, researchers at the University of California, San Francisco, found that telomeres lengthened by 10 percent in men who for five years ate a diet rich in plant foods while practicing yoga and stress management. For the men themselves, that's the equivalent of turning back the clock twenty years! By the end of the study, the men's telomerase levels had increased, too. By contrast, the twenty-five men in a control group (who did not follow the same diet and lifestyle guidelines) had a 3 percent shortening of their cells' telomeres over five years.

Telomeres, Aging, and Weight Loss

In my practice as a dietitian and DASH expert, I've found that when my clients follow my DASH Diet Younger You plan, they get visibly younger. One big reason is weight loss. They shed weight on a plant-focused diet, almost effortlessly and automatically. That's because plant foods are naturally more satisfying. Barbara Rolls's research at the Pennsylvania State University demonstrated that foods high in water and fiber, namely fruits and vegetables, are bulky and filling, and they slow the absorption of nutrients, so that you feel full sooner and longer. Further, the calories on a plant-based diet are relatively low for the quantity of food that you get to eat. There's no need to even worry about calories when you make fruits and vegetables the foundation of your diet. The fiber, heart-healthy fats, nuts, and seeds on a plant-based diet slow the entire digestion process, which means you will be getting energy from your meals gradually, over a longer time, thus quenching your hunger for hours longer. This combination of food will help you avoid overeating, naturally. Weight loss is the net effect, which is good news for anti-aging. In fact, new research shows that losing weight (or maintaining a healthy weight) will increase telomere length.

Researchers at the University of Medicine and Dentistry of New Jersey recruited 1,122 women aged eighteen to seventy-six to test the length of their telomeres. Among them were 119 women who were obese. Using the women's white blood cells, the researchers were able to measure their telomeres. What really made a difference in the length of telomeres was the women's weight. The lean women had significantly longer telomeres; the heavy women had shorter telomeres. Staying lean and in shape seems to have a long-range protective effect against aging.

Either losing weight or staying at a healthy weight can be a miracle when it comes to turning back the clock. After all, excess weight makes us older in so many ways. It strains our joints and aggravates back pain. It leads to fatty liver and gallbladder problems. It increases our risks for several types of cancer, diabetes, heart disease, and strokes. All of these problems add up to one thing: an older body.

But not anymore—now you have a plan that will make you healthier and younger! If you're like most people, you've chalked aging up to "bad genes," and you've concluded there's nothing you can do about it. But your genes, and your telomeres, are not necessarily your fate. As science shows, telomeres lengthen to the degree that you change how you eat and live. So for anyone in the wrong end of the gene pool, fruits, vegetables, and other plant foods may be the best youth preserver around.

DASH Wrinkles Now: 7 Skin-Friendly Fruits and Vegetables

The wrong diet can have a devastating effect on one of the largest and most important organs in your body: skin. One sign of poor skin care habits is the premature appearance of fine lines and wrinkles, something that can add years to your age. Fight wrinkles with the following skin-friendly fruits and vegetables:

Avocados. This fruit is high in healthy fats that reduce skin inflamm-aging. Inflammation is a leading cause of aging, including premature aging of the skin.

Blueberries. These are packed with powerful antioxidants called polyphenols that help prevent skin aging.

Carrots. This vegetable, along with other orange-pigmented veggies, is packed with carotenoids. Studies show that people with naturally high levels of carotenoids in their skin have fewer wrinkles and fewer signs of sun damage. That's because over time, these antioxidants set up camp in your skin. When they do that, they begin to act as a natural sunscreen to protect your skin from sun damage.

Citrus Fruits. These foods are packed with vitamin C. Although you may have considered vitamin C helpful for treating colds and flu, it can also help restore your skin in any number of ways. First, it's an essential building block for the skin-tightening protein, collagen. It's also involved in the formation of the skin's lipid layer, which helps make your skin dewy and moist. With vitamin C, there's hope for improving wrinkles. A 2007 study published in *the American Journal of Clinical Nutrition* recruited more than 4,000 women between the ages of forty and seventy-four to see how their vitamin C intake affected the skin aging process. It turned out that women who ate more foods rich in vitamin C had smoother skin, with very few wrinkles. Some of the best sources of vitamin C are fruits such as oranges, grapefruit, strawberries, guava, and papaya.

Kale. Like other greens, kale is full of an antioxidant called lutein that helps protect against oxid-aging. Kale is also a rich

(continued)

23

source of iron, which helps oxygenate your skin, and of beta-carotene (pro-vitamin A), which helps prevent untimely aging.

Red Bell Peppers. This veggie is loaded with beta-carotene and vitamin E; both help retain moisture in the skin.

Tomatoes. These contain lycopene, a skin-friendly antioxidant that also cuts the risk of cancer. Cooked tomatoes release more lycopene than raw ones do.

Plants Fight Oxid-Aging

The rate at which we age or don't age also corresponds to the antioxidant content of what we eat. Certain vitamins, minerals, and other substances work as antioxidants by preventing the oxidation, or "rusting," of living tissues by free radicals. The best-known antioxidant team is composed of the vitamins A, C, and E and the mineral selenium. You obtain these and other antioxidants from fruits, vegetables, seeds, nuts, and, to a lesser extent, whole grains. The body produces its own natural antioxidants, too, and along with dietary antioxidants, they help prevent cell and tissue damage. An article in *Annals of the New York Academy of Sciences* from 2006 pointed out that the addition of antioxidants to the diet can increase the average life span—perhaps by five years.

What foods are the highest in antioxidants? Here's a brief list: strawberries, raspberries, red plums, red and green cabbage, grapefruits, oranges, spinach, broccoli, green grapes, onions, peas, apples, cauliflower, tomatoes, peaches, leeks, bananas, and lettuce. All of these foods—and more—are part of the DASH Diet Younger You plan. It's loaded with antioxidant-rich foods that will keep you young and vibrant.

At the same time, you'll be minimizing foods that promote

free radical damage, namely red meat and pork. Red meats are high in iron, which is easily oxidized (remember the rusting analogy). The fats in pork are very susceptible to turning rancid, either in the fridge or in your body. Eat too much iron or fats that are prone to rancidity, and your body starts generating more free radicals.

I'm not saying you have to give up red meat and pork on the DASH Diet Younger You plan—not at all. Both have benefits, including protein and a cornucopia of minerals. But you want to avoid eating too much of them. If you eat these foods occasionally, you can take advantage of the nutrients they offer without worrying about their causing free radical damage. This plan recommends that you eat these foods no more than two or three times a week. That way, you automatically minimize the production of free radicals.

A diet richer in the plant foods is a simple way to allow you to occasionally get the benefits of meat, if you so choose, while increasing the antioxidant content of your meals and reducing your risk of disease.

Can't I Just Pop Antioxidant Supplements?

The short answer: No!

Many people try to offset free radical damage by popping antioxidant supplements like beta-carotene and vitamins C and E. Recent research is challenging our infatuation with popping these supplements, because it may be downright dangerous. Research conducted by an international consortium, which included one of my nutrition professors at the University of Illinois at Chicago, revealed that these

(continued)

25

antioxidant supplements didn't prevent lung cancers; instead, the studies found more, albeit smaller, tumors in smokers who took them. And the once highly touted vitamin E supplements may actually worsen heart disease.

A 2014 article published in the prestigious *Annals of Internal Medicine* said this: "The U.S. Preventive Services Task Force recommends against the use of beta-carotene or vitamin E supplements for the prevention of cardiovascular disease or cancer." So useless are the supplements, say the scientists, that we should not waste time even studying them.

The take-home message here for all of us: Get your antioxidants from plant foods, not pills!

Did You Say You Hate Vegetables?

We need to talk.

I've always been a "plant chick." Not only do I like to eat fruits and vegetables, I really love growing them, too. I've recently been harvesting broccoli, cherry tomatoes, romaine, and Swiss chard. My lemon, lime, and grapefruit trees are in bloom. As I write this, my home-grown sugar pea pods and cabbage are almost ready to eat. Getting my hands in the dirt, planting veggies, and harvesting my dinner "for free" are exciting for me. Fresh home-grown veggies are so much tastier, as well as being richer in antioxidants than those you find sitting on the store shelves. How fun to come home from work with no idea of what to make for dinner, but then to be inspired to create something new and delicious by the array of fresh herbs and veggies in your own garden.

Okay, so you might not like vegetables as much as I do. As a reformed veggie hater, I've got some suggestions for you to help you overcome your veggie phobia and pump up the veggies in your (and your family's) diet:

- Add shredded carrots and zucchini, or other finely chopped vegetables, to pasta sauce, cook, and serve it over your favorite pasta. (Or cook grated carrots or zucchini for a couple of minutes in boiling water, and use that instead of pasta. Sometimes I will serve the sauce over green beans or broccoli, and it is fabulous!)
- Top enchiladas, tacos, salads, or grilled chicken or fish with vegetable-based salsas, such as my Texas Caviar (page 186).
- Make kebabs. Skewer chunks of tomato, onion, zucchini, and chicken on kebab sticks; brush with extra virgin olive oil, sprinkle with an Italian herb mix, grill, and serve.
- Purée vegetables such as carrots or broccoli and add them to soup stock for a creamy soup. Soup is very filling. It can help tame your appetite so you eat less at meals.
- Add grated zucchini or carrots to muffins and breads.
- Make your own pizza. Top it with tomatoes, onions, bell peppers, broccoli, mushrooms, and other vegetables.
- Slip sprouts, slices of tomato, or leaves of lettuce into sandwiches and wraps. Use mashed avocado or hummus as a spread instead of mayonnaise.
- Try the baby versions. In some veggies, the flavors intensify as they mature. If you're put off by the sometimes strong or bitter tastes of cruciferous and green vegetables, try eating baby vegetables instead. They're usually milder and less bitter than their mature counterparts. Experiment with baby spinach, baby kale, baby Brussels sprouts, and other baby vegetables. You might just find yourself loving the vegetables you think you hate.

- Roast them. Roasting caramelizes the natural sugars in veggies and often changes the perspective of die-hard veggie haters. Serve roasted vegetables to your family and see them eat their words (and veggies!).
- Dip 'em. Snack on raw, cut-up veggies, dipping them in your favorite salsa or salad dressings. Many veggies taste milder and sweeter when raw. See the recipe section (Chapter 8) for suggestions on healthy, tasty dips.

Simply use your ingenuity, and I predict you'll be a vegetable lover in no time—and a younger-looking one at that!

I DASHed Aging!

I did not like vegetables. But after reading up on what they could do for me and consulting Marla, I decided to give them a second chance. I was motivated, too, because I had developed metabolic syndrome, which can lead to diabetes. I weighed 225 pounds when I started, and my triglycerides were dangerously high at 978. My blood pressure was 189/104, very scary. I learned that all of these bad numbers are a sign of rapid interior aging.

I started the DASH Diet Younger You plan and learned how to replace a lot of the meat meals I was eating with plant proteins. Week by week, I started gradually eating more vegetables. After five months on the plan, health miracles happened. I got my weight down to 184 pounds. My triglycerides dipped to a healthy 95. And my blood pressure is now 118/72, without medication. I believe this plan saved my health and my life.

—Jane W.

Focus on Good Plant Oils, Too

By now, most of us are savvy enough to steer clear of nasty hydrogenated oils (aka trans fats) and saturated fats that can gum up arteries, cause cell damage, elevate levels of LDL ("bad") cholesterol, and increase your risk of heart attack.

But there are other fats to push out of your diet, too. Ironically, some of these are vegetable oils, namely soy, flaxseed, and corn oils. All three are very susceptible to oxidation, which can turn them into toxic chemicals, either during storage or in your body, that will generate free radicals. They can also trigger chronic inflammation, increasing your risk for arthritis, which can be more problematic as you age, and certainly could make you feel older. If you do use these oils on occasion, store them in your refrigerator—or just avoid them altogether.

There are other plant oils I don't recommend. One is coconut oil. Coconut oil has become trendy of late, but despite what you may have read in new "research," it is pure saturated fat and thus will help your body produce unneeded excess cholesterol. Saturated fats are also implicated in inflammation and may increase the risk of diabetes. Unfortunately, you'll continue to see more coconut oil in processed foods as a replacement for hydrogenated vegetable oils (with their trans fats), because it is light-flavored and works well to produce crunchy or crisp fried foods and pastries.

I don't recommend palm oil, either, for similar reasons. Traditional cultures (such as on many Pacific islands and in areas of Southeast Asia) where coconut and palm oils are staples have higher rates of obesity, diabetes, and heart disease.

What are good choices for plant-sourced oils? My favorites for healthy aging are olive oil, peanut oil, and canola oil. Extra virgin olive oil, in particular, is a monounsaturated fat rich in vitamin E.

Keep these oils in your refrigerator, since they also can turn rancid, especially if you, like me, rarely use them. Extra virgin olive oil is best for sautéing and for salad dressings. Peanut oil can be used for higher-temperature stir-frying. And canola oil is a neutral-flavored oil that can be used in almost any type of cooking. Look for canola oil that has not been genetically modified (non-GMO), since we do not yet know what the process of genetic engineering does to our health. Peanut oil and extra virgin olive oil are non-GMO foods.

Other good sources of anti-aging fats include avocados and nuts, especially walnuts and almonds.

Finally, DASH to Longevity

While I was designing the DASH Diet Younger You plan, I wanted to know what effect it might have on longevity. Could it help us live longer?

For the answer, I looked to research on longevity and the vegetarian lifestyle. After all, my new plan is largely vegetarian, with its focus on fruits and vegetables. Happily, I found mounds of research showing that vegetarians do live longer than meat-eaters. And one very recent study caught my eye. Published in 2013 in *JAMA Internal Medicine*, the study recruited more than 73,000 men and women in their mid- to upper fifties who were cancer free and heart disease free at the start of the study. The participants were Seventh-Day Adventists, many of whom follow a mostly vegetarian diet. Vegetarians made up roughly half of the group. It included the full gamut of vegetarians: vegans, who eat only plant foods; lacto-ovo vegetarians, who include eggs and dairy products in their diet; pesco-vegetarians, who also consume seafood; and semivegetarians, who shun red meat but may eat chicken and fish.

The people in this study had typically been vegetarians for nineteen to thirty-nine years. Over a six-year period, only 2,570 of the participants died, or about 4 percent. Vegans, lacto-ovo vegetarians, and pesco-vegetarians had the lowest death rates. All the vegetarians were fairly lean, not overweight or obese, and rarely suffered from any diseases of aging, such as high blood pressure and heart disease.

Clearly, the survival edge came primarily from plant-focused eating. So unless your aging plans include obesity and other lifestyle-related health problems, it's time to switch to the DASH Diet Younger You plan. It's the way to a long, healthy life.

CHAPTER 3

Brighten Your Plate with the Colors of Youth

When you choose plant foods for their anti-aging benefits, think color: red, orange, yellow, green, blue, purple, even white. All of these colors indicate that the food is full of flavonoids, pigments that tint the food. But flavonoids do more than that. They're powerful anti-aging substances that work wonders for good health and longevity, in many different ways.

For instance, flavonoids stimulate collagen growth and produce firmer skin cells with fewer lines and wrinkles. They help prevent degenerative and inflammatory conditions and can help repair DNA (as we age, our DNA begins to degrade). Some flavonoids can even lengthen telomeres.

Flavonoids fight oxid-aging, too. As antioxidants, they neutralize free radicals, those nasty molecules capable of damaging cells and increasing disease risk. Flavonoids boost brainpower, too; recent research suggests they may be able to slow or reverse age-related memory loss.

Some flavonoids help the body produce nitric oxide (NO), which dilates your blood vessels, thus lowering blood pressure and improving blood flow to all parts of your body, including your skin. You'll want to say YES to having more NO in your system, since flavonoids can increase your natural supply of this internal fountain of youth at the cellular level.

Other flavonoids are cancer fighters. They work by causing cell death (apoptosis) in cancer cells. They also appear to foster cell death in cells where there is already genetic damage that could initiate cancer. What's more, they help eliminate toxins that can cause cancer.

There are more than five thousand flavonoids in foods, and most have hard-to-pronounce names. Don't worry, you don't have to remember any of the names or types of all these plant chemicals. Just learn their color categories, and you'll see how powerful certain fruits and vegetables can be in keeping you youthful, beautiful, and healthy.

Color Yourself Young

Different color groups of fruits and vegetables contain different flavonoids. Therefore, eating a variety of colors and kinds each day gives more protection against aging and disease. Some examples:

Blue and Red-Purple

Blue and red-purple fruits and vegetables are full of anthocyanins and polyphenols. These flavonoids fight free radicals, carcinogens, and aging in general. Anthocyanins, in particular, help normalize blood sugar and iron out wrinkles by promoting healthy collagen in your skin.

One of the best sources of anthocyanins and polyphenols is berries. I adore berries and can't get enough of them. The red-purple color that tints strawberries, raspberries, and blueberries, along with the stone fruits, like plums and cherries, is so good for us.

The anthocyanins and other phenolic compounds found in berries may reduce the ability of blood cells to form dangerous blood clots, make the linings of our veins and arteries younger, lower bad cholesterol, and reduce inflammation. They literally make us younger from the inside out.

If you think heart disease and faster aging are just "in the cards" for you, based on your family history, you're in for a surprise. These flavonoids change the way your genes work and can turn off the genes that make bad things happen. Research has shown that they can reduce the risk of blood clots, independent of lowering cholesterol. This means that your risk of a stroke or a heart attack is lowered—just by eating more fruits and vegetables.

To get these benefits, eat:

- Blueberries
- Blackberries
- Purple grapes
- Cherries
- Plums
- Red cabbage
- Eggplant

Green

Green fruits and vegetables provide flavonoids with antioxidant properties that protect our cells from cancer-causing agents and reduce the risk of heart disease. Dark-green leafy vegetables such as spinach, collard greens, kale, and romaine provide two flavonoids—lutein and zeaxanthin—that may help keep your eyes young and protect against some cancers.

Since ancient times, tea leaves have been used to foretell the future. Well, if you've been sipping a lot of green tea lately, those leaves might just portend a long life for you. That's because regular drinkers of green tea live longer. In one 1992 study, researchers examined the link between green tea consumption and longevity by following the lives of 3,380 Japanese women for nine years. The women who drank the most green tea—several cups daily—lived many years longer than the other women. The researchers suggested that green tea protects against premature death.

But how? The answer probably lies in green tea's polyphenols, such as epigallocatechin gallate. Polyphenols are powerful antioxidants. In fact, the polyphenols in green tea are even more powerful than the more well-known powerhouse of antioxidants, vitamin E. My advice: Live long and prosper by drinking green tea daily.

In addition to enjoying green tea, populate your diet with these longevity boosters:

- Green peas
- Avocados
- Green grapes
- Honeydew melons
- Kiwifruit
- Broccoli
- Green beans
- Brussels sprouts
- Dark-green leafy vegetables of all kinds

Orange and Yellow

Orange and deep-yellow fruits and vegetables are loaded with flavonoids called carotenoids. They give fruits and vegetables their distinctive yellow and orange hues.

You've probably heard folklore that carrots are good for your eyes. This isn't a myth. The beta-carotenes in carrots and sweet potatoes and the lutein and zeaxanthin in spinach, kale, sweet corn, and romaine help prevent cataracts and age-related macular degeneration, two major causes of visual impairment as we get older.

You'll find all these powerful flavonoids in these foods:

Beta-carotene

- Apricots
- Peaches
- Cantaloupe
- Mangoes
- Oranges
- Tangerines
- Sweet potatoes
- Carrots
- Winter squash
- Pumpkin

Lutein and Zeaxanthin

- Spinach
- Kale
- Swiss chard
- Peas
- Kiwifruit
- Brussels sprouts
- Broccoli
- Sweet corn

"Rutin" Out Spider Veins

Wrinkles aren't the only visible signs of aging. Those spider veins and varicose veins road-mapping over your legs are another reminder that you're getting on in years. Fortunately, you can defy these signs of aging, without having vein surgery.

For background, spider veins and varicose veins are most often caused by the gradual weakening and deterioration of capillaries. The capillaries, because they're so small, get bullied by free radicals. The tiny vessels then rupture and bleed, showing up on the surface of your legs as broken veins.

Rutin, a flavonoid found naturally in fruits and vegetables, such as citrus fruits, apples, cranberries, and peaches, safeguards capillaries in a couple of different ways. For one thing, it improves circulation. It can also protect the potency of vitamin C so that it can fend off free radicals and maintain the production of youth-giving collagen. After eating more rutin-rich foods, you'll say good-bye to ugly veins and hello to younger-looking legs.

Red

Red fruits and vegetables are rich in lycopene (tomatoes, for example) or anthocyanins (raspberries, for example). Both types of flavonoids are believed to promote heart health, improve your memory, protect against bladder infections, and lower the risk of some types of cancers.

Include the following "reds" in your diet:

- Cherries
- Watermelon

- Cranberries
- Pink grapefruits
- Strawberries
- Red bell peppers
- Tomatoes (the lycopene in tomatoes is more easily absorbed when the tomatoes are cooked or canned)

Uncork This Red Anti-Aging Flavonoid

Found in grape skins and red wine, resveratrol is a potent flavonoid that can help prevent heart disease, stroke damage, and some cancers. And it has been shown to extend the life span of certain cells.

Resveratrol works its anti-aging magic by increasing the activity in the body of a certain enzyme called SIR2. In turn, SIR2 guards the DNA in cells. The more you protect your DNA, the more slowly you age.

DASH to Color

For all the amazing benefits of these colorful foods, how many fruits and vegetables do you need to eat each day? Most health authorities advocate at least five servings a day—an amount you'll surpass on the DASH Diet Younger You plan. Key to the DASH diet is having at least four or five servings of vegetables and three to five servings of fruit each day. And you'll have a lot of variety, too. That's the best way to get the most from colorful (and white) foods. I'm a big fan of eating a variety of whole foods, rather than singling out a few "superfoods." It's hard to think of any fruits and vegetables that aren't good for you, especially now that we know they're so potent against aging.

Red Wine Mask

Not a wine drinker? Here's a way to harness the anti-aging benefits of resveratrol, externally, with an easy-to-make facial mask. Applied three to four times a week, this mask will help make your skin appear more youthful and firm by minimizing fine lines and wrinkles. The sugar provides a great exfoliant to eat away dead skin cells, and the honey has anti-germ properties that pull out pore-clogging bacteria and debris. Also, the egg white has a tightening effect.

Ingredients:

- 1 egg white

- 3 tablespoons red wine

- 2 tablespoons honey

- 1 tablespoon table sugar

Directions:

Combine all the ingredients in a small mixing bowl and whisk together. Spread the paste gently and evenly on your face with your fingertips. Lie down on your back, relax, and leave the mask on for a half hour. Then rinse it off with warm water and pat dry with a clean towel. Apply a moisturizer to seal in your skin's natural moisture.

White Plant Foods Can Be Healthy, Too!

Don't reject white foods wholesale. Just because they don't produce a visible color doesn't mean they're unhealthy. In general, white fruits and veggies promote heart health and beneficial cholesterol levels, lower the risk of some cancers, and fight aging. A few examples:

Apples. This fruit is packed with quercetin, lots of soluble fiber and roughage (insoluble fiber), and antioxidants, including vitamin C.

Cauliflower. This cruciferous vegetable is rich in vitamin C, potassium, fiber, folate, and the phytochemical isothiocyanate, which has disease-fighting properties.

Nuts. Just about every nut known to humankind is a rich source of inflammation-fighting flavonoids. Topping the list are almonds, walnuts, pecans, and Brazil nuts. A single Brazil nut contains exactly the right amount of selenium, a powerful antioxidant, to meet your daily need and fight oxid-aging.

Onions. These veggies provide organosulfur compounds, which are powerful antioxidants; allyl sulfides, which can reduce blood pressure and tumor formation; quercetin, which is anti-inflammatory; and saponins, which can reduce tumors and cho-lesterol. Quercetin deserves an honorable mention here, because it improves lung function. In studies, people who eat a diet rich in quercetin-containing fruits and vegetables are less likely to suffer from asthma. Plus, as seen in studies of people in Asia, they have much lower rates of lung cancer.

Potatoes. These are chock-full of vitamin C and potassium, a good source of fiber and several B vitamins. Just go easy on the portion sizes, especially if you're trying to drop pounds or if you have issues with blood sugar control, since potatoes can spike glucose.

DASH Wrinkles: The Power of Quercetin

Quercetin, found in onions and apples, has real power against wrinkles. Under normal conditions, skin cells replicate; that is, they make copies of themselves just like you'd make copies of documents. As long as the replication process goes along without trouble, your skin stays supple and young. But if the replication process breaks down and skin cells stop replicating, your skin loses elasticity and collagen. The result is wrinkly, saggy skin.

Quercetin to the rescue: One 2004 study showed that when quercetin and rutin were added to nonreplicating (dying) skin cells, the cells came back to life and began to reproduce again. You can prevent the problem in the first place by eating foods rich in this antioxidant. Quercetin can also help bump up the production of skin-firming collagen and protect the skin's resident antioxidants from destruction by UVA rays. For younger-looking skin, eat quercetin-loaded fruits and veggies. You'll glow from within!

CHAPTER 4

Detox with a Healthy Microbiota

In the early 1900s, a Russian microbiologist, Elie Metchnikoff, was studying the aging process while working at the Pasteur Institute in Paris. He observed that the longest-lived people in the world were the Hunzas of Kashmir, the Georgians in Eastern Europe, and the Bulgarians. The latter had an unusually long life span for the early 1900s, with an average life expectancy of eighty-seven years, and four out of every thousand lived past 100 years of age.

What was their secret? Metchnikoff identified a common denominator in the diets of all three of these peoples: They regularly ate large amounts of fermented milks—yogurt, kefir, and sour milk—all containing beneficial organisms. Metchnikoff believed that the aging process was related to a healthy balance of these good bacteria ("probiotics") in the gut.

And he was mostly right, despite frequent opposition to his theory during his lifetime. Today, there's been an explosion of research as scientists learn more about the benefits of probiotics: good digestion, effective detoxification, a stronger immune system at any age, and, of course, increased longevity.

You Are What You Host

You have trillions of bacteria living in your gut, known collectively as a microbiota. I know this sounds bad, but it's actually good. Most of these "bugs" are beneficial, and they do a lot for us. When you have a healthy microbiota, the "good bugs" (bacteria associated with good intestinal health) crowd out most "bad bugs," which can include *Candida albicans* (yeast) and *E. coli* (which is found in all intestines but certain strains can cause illness if excess comes in from contaminated foods). Take a look (the list is long!). Probiotics are known to:

- Maintain a healthy digestive system. This is something you want, since untreated digestive problems can become chronic, compromising your immune system and triggering other serious illnesses.
- Protect against "leaky gut syndrome," a condition in which the intestinal lining is damaged by a poor diet, infection, or medications, allowing germs or toxins to leak through the intestinal walls to contaminate the bloodstream. Intact food proteins can also leak through, which can lead to development of food allergies.
- Assist our bodies in making vitamins, including thiamine, riboflavin, vitamin B6, and vitamin K.
- Fight off and crowd out dangerous organisms in the intestines, including *Escherichia coli* (*E. coli*) strains that are pathogens known to cause severe diarrhea and can be potentially fatal.

- Reduce the risk of infection and boost immunity.
- Suppress inflammation that leads to digestive diseases, such as Crohn's disease, irritable bowel syndrome (IBS), and ulcerative colitis.
- Break down phytochemicals from foods so the body can absorb them. Many phytochemicals provide an anti-aging benefit.
- Promote bone density by helping the body absorb important bone-building minerals. Good bone density is a sign of youthfulness.
- Prevent becoming overweight or obesity. Research has shown that the transplantation of good "bugs" from the guts of lean rats into the guts of obese rats causes them to lose weight, without a change in diet. Incidentally, people who are obese have more bad bugs in their gut than lean people have. People who follow a plant-focused diet are more likely to have more of the beneficial bacteria, which helps keep them lean.
- Help control appetite by regulating the production of leptin, the fullness hormone.
- Help reverse type 2 diabetes by normalizing blood sugar levels. It is suspected that changes in gut microbiota may explain reversal of diabetes after bariatric (obesity) surgery.
- Can help slash the risk of colon cancer and some types of breast cancer. Probiotics neutralize dangerous enzymes that convert potential cancer-causing agents to full-blown carcinogens.
- Improve your mood. Beneficial bacteria help produce brain chemicals that ease feelings of anxiety and depression. More serotonin (the happy hormone) is produced in your gut than in your brain. Bad bacteria, on the other hand, may actually trigger anxiety and depression.

Few nutritional agents do so much, at so many different levels, as the good bugs. One reason you'll feel so good after you start this plan is that you'll be nourishing yourself with these microbiotic do-gooders.

But When Things Go Wrong...

Normally, you have mostly good bugs in your gut. But if bad bugs overwhelm the good ones, you can get sick. Bad bugs can produce gas, bloating, and diarrhea. They can interfere with nutrient absorption and cross into the bloodstream, causing septicemia, a serious life-threatening infection that can worsen very quickly. Diseases caused by an overgrowth of bad bacteria include inflammatory bowel disease, some types of cancer, and cardiovascular disease. Allergies, asthma, and even obesity are also related to an imbalance of intestinal bacteria.

What causes this imbalance? A major trigger is a poor diet (a typical American diet is one example), since the food we eat helps determine what kinds of bacteria can thrive in our gut. A 2012 study of older people looked into this.

Researchers at University College Cork in Ireland studied elderly people who were living in nursing homes or assisted living, as well as seniors who lived in their own homes. Some big differences emerged. The people who lived at home tended to have a rich diversity of healthy bacteria in their guts. The reason, said the researchers, was that those seniors had high-fiber diets. They ate mostly fruits, vegetables, and a range of grains—exactly the type of diet that feeds healthy bacteria, and the type of diet you'll be eating on the DASH Diet Younger You plan.

By contrast, the people who lived in nursing homes had guts that were overrun with bad bacteria. Those seniors ate a lot of processed, high-starch and high-sugar foods like mashed potatoes, porridge, sweetened tea, puddings, and biscuits or cookies. A diet like this—rich in added sugars and starch and low in fiber—is a recipe for disaster because it feeds the growth of bad bacteria and yeast.

Too much meat does the same. A growing body of studies affirms that people who eat a lot of meat have an unbalanced microbiota, compared to those on a predominantly plant-based diet. Meat contains an amino acid called carnitine. In the gut, carnitine is broken down into trimethylamine (TMA), which is later converted to trimethylamine-N-oxide (TMAO) by the liver, with gut bacteria playing a major role. The more TMAO you have in your blood, the higher your risk of heart attack, stroke, and death. Researchers speculate that TMAO prevents the cleanup of cholesterol from plaque deposits in the arteries, creating a condition known as atherosclerosis. This may be one reason vegetarians have a heart health advantage. Since they don't consume meat, they have little or none of the gut bacteria that converts carnitine to TMAO.

A diet rich in simple sugars is harmful, too. Fructose from honey, sweetened beverages, and the HFCS (high-fructose corn syrup) found in most commercially baked goods and added-sugar food products fuels rapid growth of bad bacteria. And, of course, this is differentiated from the fructose from fruit, since that comes packaged with lots of fiber, especially the soluble fiber that slows its absorption and helps nourish good bacteria.

Another fascinating observation from research is that people living in Asia tend to have a healthier microbiota than Americans and other Westernized people. Asian diets, of course, are low in meat and very high in plant foods, including fermented probiotic plant foods, such as kimchi in Korea and miso and tempeh in Japan. On the other hand, Western diets are loaded with meat, saturated fats, sugar, and refined starches—all known to inflame the gut.

Beyond bad nutrition, other causes of an unhealthy gut are

environmental factors, such as pollution and the excessive prescribing and use of antibiotics. Antibiotics are notorious for annihilating bacteria—including the good ones. If your physician has put you on antibiotics, you should definitely consider adding probiotic foods like yogurt and kefir to your diet to prevent opportunistic bad bacteria and yeast from taking over and to repopulate the gut with healthy bacteria. Aging is often characterized by a shift in the balance of your gut microbiota toward a higher population of bad bugs.

When you put this whole picture together, you'll discover how important a plant-focused, whole food diet like DASH is—and how it keeps your gastrointestinal tract younger and healthier the older you get. That means better overall health and slower aging in your golden years.

Detoxing with DASH: Populating Your Gut with Good Guys

Once you start the DASH Diet Younger You plan, your body will undergo a natural, ongoing detox that will help you feel and look young. Unlike highly publicized detoxes, there's no rigorous fasting, starving, or cleansing with questionable ingredients—just delicious pure food filled with probiotics and a class of foods called prebiotics. Prebiotics are nondigestible fibers that remain in the digestive tract, where they feed and stimulate the growth of beneficial bacteria. Put another way, they are food for probiotics via fermentation in the gut.

Here's how it works:

The DASH Diet Younger You plan includes probiotic foods for a healthy gut microbiota. The best-known probiotic foods are yogurt and other fermented dairy products. New research reveals that the probiotics in these foods do not actually colonize your gut; rather, they pass genetic material to the good bacteria in your intestines, and in doing so, improve the mix of healthy bacteria. Among these healthy bacteria are *Lactobacillus bulgaricus*, *Lactobacillus acidophilus*, *Bifidobacterium bifidus*, and *Streptococcus thermophilus*.

These bacteria work by fermenting the milk sugar lactose and turning it into lactic acid. People who have trouble digesting lactose often find that they can tolerate these fermented dairy foods much more easily than milk. For a long time, I couldn't drink milk without having severe intestinal pain. After yogurt companies introduced tastier, light yogurts, I jumped on the bandwagon. Surprisingly, I then found that my milk intolerance disappeared. I'm convinced that the good bacteria from the yogurt improved my ability to digest milk.

I DASHed Aging!

At sixty-four years old, I had lots of digestive issues, including heartburn and constipation. I just felt fatigued all the time, and I couldn't seem to lose weight. DASH was my next step. I stayed on the plan religiously and made sure to eat probiotic and prebiotic foods daily. In only six weeks on the DASH program, I lost fifteen pounds and dropped my blood pressure from 157/88 to 106/62, without medication. I have not needed any of my heartburn meds since starting the plan. My system is running regularly again, and I have the energy of someone half my age.

—*Patty N.*

In addition to adding good bugs to your diet, you also want to nourish them. This is where prebiotics come in. As explained earlier, prebiotics are foods you eat that help promote the growth of the healthy gut bacteria.

Sources of prebiotics include fruits, legumes, and whole grains.

Besides boosting your levels of prebiotics, these foods do other good deeds, such as normalizing levels of cholesterol, triglycerides, and blood sugar. Great sources of the nourishing prebiotics include almonds, bananas, chicory, asparagus, onions, garlic, oregano, artichokes, leeks, jicama, and many other fiber-rich plant foods.

One set of superior prebiotics are fructooligosaccharides (FOS). FOS are fermented in the gut by the healthy bacteria. They have an impressive list of benefits: They improve the absorption of minerals, including calcium; reduce levels of bad cholesterol and triglycerides; and improve regularity. FOS are found in many foods, including bananas, onions, garlic, and asparagus. You can also find FOS supplements, but the point of DASH is not to pop supplements, it's to eat foods that naturally provide healthy nutrients.

Found in artichokes and other veggies, inulin is another excellent prebiotic. It nourishes the probiotic *Bifidobacterium* species, which are known to be associated with a healthy gut.

Eating probiotics and prebiotics puts your body into a natural ongoing detox state so that you're always in "rejuvenation" mode and less likely to be sidelined by illness. Nurturing the healthy gut microbiota allows your gut to be "cleansed" the natural way.

DASH Wrinkles: How Probiotics Help

When it comes to wrinkles, your worst enemy is the sun. It hits your skin with harmful ultraviolet rays. Over time, those rays gradually disintegrate collagen and elastin, the two main proteins in skin, causing saggy skin, wrinkles, and premature skin aging. Because of this damage, dermatologists have long recommended that we wear sunscreen—not just to prevent wrinkles but also to protect against skin cancer.

(continued)

Emerging research now affirms that consuming probiotics may act as an "internal sunscreen." In 2009, French researchers revealed that they had discovered that when skin cells were exposed to a high level of ultraviolet light, then fed the probiotic *Lactobacillus johnsonii*, the cells recovered from the UV damage. It's not clear why there was such a powerful benefit, but it appears that consuming probiotics may exert sun protection systemically. Quite possibly, this means that the probiotics enter the body and are delivered to skin tissues, where they do their protective work.

Other studies have shown that probiotics help manage atopic dermatitis, a type of eczema that causes itching and inflammation. Clearly, probiotics are skin-friendly organisms.

Fiber 101

You don't want to turn your nose up at fruits and vegetables. Another big reason: They're high in fiber. Fiber is an all-inclusive name for a variety of carbohydrates in foods that do not, by themselves, provide nutrients but do greatly affect the way your body absorbs and uses nutrients.

In general, high-fiber foods help keep a healthy gut. Some types of fiber are fermented in the gut, a breakdown process that produces beneficial short-chain acids. These acids nourish the cells of the gut and help prevent intestinal permeability, or leakage. "Leaky gut" is tied to increased inflammation and an overactive immune system that can produce allergies and autoimmune diseases, in which the body's own cells mistake body tissues for foreign invaders.

There are two main types of fiber: soluble and insoluble. Insoluble fiber, which is also referred to as roughage, helps to keep waste moving through the intestinal tract. Soluble fiber thickens the liquid digested food (chyme) so that we absorb the nutrients slowly, thus getting energy over a longer time and keeping hunger at bay. Soluble fiber absorbs some fat and cholesterol and helps escort it out of the body. It draws water out of the intestinal lining, keeping your waste softer, as well as bulkier, and therefore easier to move through the intestines.

Some of the best sources of soluble and insoluble fiber are fruits, which is why I encourage people to eat their fruits instead of drinking them. Juicing removes all that fabulous fiber from fruits (or pulverizes it), so you're missing out if you reach for OJ instead of the whole orange. Fiberful fruits are full of prebiotics that nourish the good bacteria of the gut.

How much fiber should we include in our diet? Most dietitians suggest about 14 grams of fiber for every 1,000 calories in our diet. If you have an intestinal disease, such as irritable bowel syndrome (IBS), ulcerative colitis, Crohn's disease, or diverticulosis, consult your physician and/or dietitian before radically changing your diet and increasing your fiber intake. And don't forget to get enough water, or you could become constipated even with more fiber. Water plumps up the fiber to help it do its job.

The bottom line is: Be nice to your colon and make it a point to eat fibrous grains, vegetables, and fruit daily. That should keep the bacteria in your gut healthy.

Listen to Your Gut

When you consider the power of probiotics and prebiotics, the old saying "gut feeling" takes on new meaning. We are learning so much about how the gut influences our thoughts, moods, aging, immunity, and even whether or not we will be overweight. If you have a gut feeling that your health isn't all it could be, or you feel old before your time, make sure you're eating probiotics and prebiotics. They can impact just about everything in your body, including how well you age.

Should You Take Supplemental Probiotics?

I prefer that you get your probiotics from food and that you enrich your microbiota from a plant-focused diet like the DASH Diet Younger You plan. But if you're considering probiotic supplements, seek advice from a health professional. There are many confusing products out there, and it's difficult to know whether their label claims accurately reflect what's inside the bottle or package. If you end up taking probiotics as a supplement, don't look at that as a cure-all. You benefit only if the probiotic is combined with a healthful diet on the whole. You can't continue to eat lots of meat, sugar, and fast food, then pop a probiotic supplement and expect a miraculous return to health.

CHAPTER 5

Kick Out Bad Sugars

Forget about being made of sugar and spice and everything nice. The truth is, sugar is aging and promotes weight gain. By the same token, cutting down on refined sugar will not only trim your body, it will also make you more youthful.

Sugar is definitely a weakness for many of us. Imagine 150 bags of sugar piled up in your kitchen. That's approximately the amount of sugar each person in the U.S. eats annually, on average. Clearly, we're eating much more than we need. The good news is that you don't need to let your sweet tooth sabotage your health—read on to discover why sugar is so bad for you and how the DASH Diet Younger You plan can help.

Sugar and Glyc-Aging

Okay, what's the problem with a little sugar? First of all, let's talk about the hormone insulin. When you ingest sugar from food, your blood sugar (glucose) goes up fast. In response, your pancreas churns out insulin, whose job, among other assignments, is to confiscate that sugar from your bloodstream and deliver it to cells to be used for energy.

Virtually all foods, except for fats, contain some sugar. Grains and starchy vegetables break down 100 percent into glucose, which is what we measure when we check blood sugar. Honey, agave syrup, and high-fructose corn syrup (HFCS) are composed of fructose and glucose. Fruits contain primarily fructose. Dairy foods contain lactose, another type of sugar, which breaks down into the sugars galactose and glucose. Blood sugar, then, is affected by all of these sugar-containing and sugar-creating foods.

When excess sugar lurks in the bloodstream, it randomly attaches to proteins, hormones, and cells—an unholy linkage that produces advanced glycation end products (AGEs). They cause your tissues to stiffen and lose elasticity and can damage your eyes, kidneys, nerves, and other organs. The longer you allow blood sugar levels to stay high, the more AGEs there will be in your system. This entire process is known as glycation, and when it starts aging you, it's called glyc-aging.

When you were younger, perhaps at a healthier weight, and more active, your body could easily mop up excess sugar from your bloodstream. But with increasing age, excess weight (especially belly fat), and inactivity, you can gradually lose your ability to keep your blood sugar at healthy levels. Your body may stop responding as well to insulin; thus, less glucose gains access to cells, with the exception of cells around your middle. Unfortunately, these cells, known as visceral fat, still respond very well to insulin. A lot of excess glucose gets deposited there, converted to fat, resulting in an accumulation of belly fat.

Some of that excess sugar gets soaked up by the liver. Only a limited amount of sugar can be stockpiled there, so the excess gets converted into fat, called triglycerides. Some of the triglycerides get stored in the liver (which can cause fatty liver disease, a dangerous condition that can lead to cirrhosis or liver cancer), and the rest gets pumped out into the bloodstream and shows up when you get your blood tests from your physician. Elevated triglycerides indicate that you are at higher risk for metabolic syndrome, diabetes, heart disease, and dementia, all conditions that can potentially shorten your life.

This is an especially important issue for me personally. I have a very strong family history of type 2 diabetes. My mother was a bad example of how poor blood sugar control can lead to heart attacks, strokes, kidney disease, and neuropathy. However, my very disciplined great-grandmother had diabetes for over thirty-five years, stayed healthy, and lived to be 101 years old.

So the question is: Will cutting down on sources of sugar keep you young, healthy, and slim?

Current research says yes, particularly when you cut down on "added sugars."

The Black-Hatted Villains: Added Sugars

As I mentioned above, fruits, vegetables, starches, and dairy foods all naturally contain sugar. "Added sugar" is different. This phrase refers to sugars and syrups purposely put in foods by manufacturers. Desserts, processed foods, sodas, and juice drinks are the top sources of added sugars. When you take a spoonful of table sugar and stir it into your coffee or tea, you're consuming added sugar.

Added sugar is bad for health and disastrous for aging. Here's why: When sugar is embedded naturally in fruits and vegetables, it works synergistically with vitamins, minerals, and phytonutrients to provide full nutrition, and the fiber slows its absorption. But when it's found isolated in your sugar bowl, or in a candy bar, it provides nothing of any nutritional value. In fact, sugar weakens your immune system. It impairs the ability of your white blood cells to kill bacteria, and it robs your body of vitamin C needed to fend off free radicals. For this reason, sugar is considered an immune system depressor.

Since aging does the same thing, you're only adding fuel to the aging fire by consuming added sugar. It has been linked to obesity, diabetes, high blood pressure, and heart disease. It is also addictive. The danger of added sugars is not just about tooth decay anymore.

The worst of the worst added sugars is high-fructose corn syrup (HFCS), used to sweeten everything from soft drinks to commercial baked goods. According to *The Journal of Nutrition*, HFCS accounts for as much as 40 percent of caloric sweeteners used in the United States. It has a long rap sheet of offenses.

For starters, it promotes the formation of AGEs, those nasty substances that play a role in aging. HFCS has been blamed for the rise of obesity, diabetes, and fatty liver disease in the United States, according to a comprehensive review article published in the journal *Alternative Medicine Review* in 2005. The article also pointed out that HFCS is more fat-forming than glucose or starches and usually causes greater spikes in triglycerides and sometimes in cholesterol than other carbohydrates. So if you find it difficult to shed pounds despite your best efforts, your problem may be too much added fructose in your diet. Recent studies have found that fructose very quickly converts into body fat.

Added sugar also triggers the dangerous accumulation of fat cells around your vital organs. In one study, sixteen volunteers went on a diet that included a lot of fructose. Alarmingly, this diet instigated the production of new fat cells around their hearts, livers, and other digestive organs in just *ten weeks*! That's scary, since once your body makes new fat cells, it can't get rid of them. They only shrink in response to a weight-loss program. And I have personally seen a similar consequence of high glucose intake, observing an autopsy of a man who, prior to his passing, had been on intravenous glucose for several months, which led to his internal organs becoming encased in fat.

Fructose can inflict yet more damage. A side effect of having high levels of fructose in your blood is a buildup of fructose in your corneas, which increases your risk for cataracts.

To me, the most distressing offense is the connection between HFCS and cancer. Researchers at the University of California, Los Angeles discovered that cancer cells readily use fructose to divide and multiply. Cancer cells apparently love to gobble up fructose for sustenance; I don't have to tell you that this is a bad scenario.

DASH Wrinkles: What Sugar Does to Your Face

To keep your skin healthy and wrinkle free, what you *don't eat* is as important as what you do eat. Too much added sugar, for example, can give rise to fine lines, wrinkles, and sagging of your skin. Added sugar initiates glycation in your body. It binds to the elastin and collagen fibers and leads to the degradation of these important skin proteins that are normally responsible for the elasticity and suppleness of the skin. Glycation also causes inflamm-aging, resulting in further destruction of the collagen and elastin fibers.

Large amounts of fructose are particularly unkind to your face. Fructose reacts more easily than other sugars with collagen and elastic, changing their characteristics and speeding up the wrinkling process as fast as nicotine does. So cut back on added sugar and fructose, and you'll have younger-looking skin.

Collateral Damage: Hunger and Cravings

Added sugar affects hunger in a couple of ways. Fructose, in particular, interferes with the action of a hormone called leptin. Its job is to signal the brain that we've had enough to eat and it's time to stop. Because fructose puts the hormone out of commission, we tend to eat...and eat and eat.

Also, when you eat too much sugar, blood glucose rises. Insulin is then pressed into action to get that glucose under control. In the process, insulin can often overshoot the target, removing too much sugar from your system. A vicious cycle ensues. There's a fast crash as your blood sugar plummets. You start feeling shaky, weak—and hungry for more sugar NOW. Under these circumstances, your body cannot efficiently metabolize sugar. Consequently, more AGEs are produced. It's thus important to slow the pace at which these damaging reactions occur. You can do that by easing off sugar and combining protein, fats, and carbohydrates in a way that keeps your blood sugar moderated, your energy levels stable throughout the day, and your hunger in check. The DASH Diet Younger You plan does this for you automatically.

I DASHed Aging!

I'm sixty-three. I wanted to go on a plan that would make me look younger, and that included losing weight and improving my skin. My skin was always blotchy and starting to look more wrinkly. At first, I was convinced that I couldn't live without "treats" and "substitutes." I learned that I was using a lot of artificial sweeteners and processed "diet" foods that were really just perpetuating my addiction to food, my excess weight, and my bad-looking skin. My cravings for food didn't truly subside for about two weeks, but I hung in there. Then my tastes and cravings changed. I began to appreciate the flavor of healthy food. I looked forward to "splurging" on steel-cut oats and apples! I lost nine pounds the first week and two pounds the second week. After ten weeks, I had lost twenty-six pounds. I can honestly say the most important thing DASH gave me, besides losing weight, is that I look and feel younger.

—Ken D.

Do Artificial Sweeteners Age You?

I'm not a big fan of artificial sweeteners. These include aspartame, sucralose, saccharin, acesulfame potassium, and sugar alcohols like sorbitol. Yes, they do reduce calories and help keep sugar out of the diet, but there may be some aging consequences. Some experts think artificial sweeteners can cause free radical damage in nerve cells, and free radicals promote oxid-aging.

Aspartame, a popular artificial sweetener, has been associated with joint pain, a sign of old age. What's more, for some people, these fake sweets can make you crave real sugar. Research suggests that they may trick our brains into desiring more sweet foods. Proof positive: Scientists analyzed the diet-soda-drinking habits of the participants in the San Antonio Heart Study, a quarter-century-long study conducted at the University of Texas Health Science Center at San Antonio. They found that people who guzzled more than twenty-one diet drinks a week were twice as likely to become overweight or obese as people who didn't drink diet soda.

If you want to avoid artificial sweeteners, fruit is a great source of natural sweetness and, of course, a key part of the DASH Diet Younger You Plan. You can also try noncaloric natural sweeteners such as stevia. Many other natural sweeteners are high in fructose or sucrose and thus may have an effect on premature aging. Some examples are honey, agave (both of which are high in fructose), molasses, and maple syrup. My advice is to make a plan to mostly avoid artificial sweeteners and added sugars; instead, choose fruits for sweetness. Fruit, with its fiber to help slow sugar absorption, will help quench hunger rather than stoke it.

Don't Be an Old Salt: Do a Sodium Shakedown

If you think sugar is bad for aging, salt may be just as nasty. The American Heart Association presented some startling research at its annual meeting in 2014 regarding the effect of excess salt on telomere length. The study involved 800 overweight or obese teenagers ages fourteen to eighteen. Researchers divided them into groups based on their salt intake. The high-salt group consumed 4,100 milligrams of salt (around 2½ teaspoons) a day; the low-salt group ate an average of less than 2,400 milligrams daily, or around a teaspoon a day or less.

The researchers then examined the teens' telomeres. First of all, the telomeres were shorter in overweight and obese teens but were even shorter in the high-salt group. The researchers suggested that high salt intake and obesity may act synergistically to speed up aging at the cellular level.

This study is definitely food for thought. To stop Father Time, you'll want to get your weight under control, plus cut back on your salt intake. You can do both naturally with the DASH Diet Younger You plan. Even so, here are some additional suggestions on how to slash the salt:

- Don't salt your food. Use herb and pepper blends or various herbs to spice it up.

- Cut way back or eliminate convenience foods such as frozen dinners. These often contain up to 1,500 milligrams of salt per serving.

- Limit bread. It is the number 1 source of sodium in the American diet.

- Do a salt sweep of your pantry. Toss out or donate high-sodium items such as packaged and canned foods.

- Avoid eating fast foods as much as possible. They are among the top sources of hidden salt in the diet.

Get Off Sugar with the DASH Diet Younger You Plan

If you want to live your optimal life, feeling and looking young, you have to really ease off sugar. You'll find this easy to do once you start the DASH Diet Younger You plan. It automatically and effortlessly reduces added sugar, and before long, you'll lose your sweet tooth. Here's how you'll avoid added sugar and eat healthier:

- You'll enjoy fresh fruit for dessert instead of cakes, cookies, pies, ice cream, candy, and other sweets.

- You're going to "de-fructose" your diet. You'll start by steer-
  ing clear of processed foods, including those that contain
  high-fructose corn syrup: sodas, juices, ketchup and other
  condiments, sauces, and salad dressings.

Sugar Surge: Juicing

Many people are into juicing, but this practice can bombard
your system with sugar, including too much natural fructose,
which is, of course, found in fruit. Juicing either pulverizes the
fruit fiber or removes it entirely. So the fructose from juice floods
into your bloodstream. This is not to say that a four-fluid-
ounce serving of juice at breakfast is bad. However, people
tend to have really big portions when they juice. Unlike other
sugars, fructose is metabolized entirely in the liver. But the
liver cannot store much sugar, so it turns most of the fructose
into triglycerides (blood fats). These triglycerides can contribute
to nonalcoholic fatty liver disease and raise your blood
triglycerides, which in turn lowers your good cholesterol (HDL).
Fructose inflicts oxidative stress on your body, aging you in
additional ways, and causes weight gain. It mystifies me, too,
that so many people juice to prevent or treat cancer, when
in effect, juicing feeds cancer cells with the sugar they need
to divide and proliferate, speeding their growth. Juicing also
eliminates many virtues of fruits and vegetables, namely the fiber
and additional antioxidants, and the ability to fill you up.

Please get your nutrients from fruits and vegetables that
are whole. You want the fiber for digestive health. You want
the bulk of whole foods to feel satisfied. And you want all the
anti-aging nutrients imparted by whole foods. Limit juice to no
more than four fluid ounces per day.

- You'll be eating some good fiber-rich carbs, such as legumes, unrefined cereals, and even whole grain bread. When eaten with protein and fat, these fiber-rich carbs stimulate normal, healthy glucose release.
- You'll enjoy one of the most desirable types of protein-rich foods: fish, especially salmon and tuna. Cold-water, fatty fish contain what are known as omega-3 fatty acids. They have been shown to work all kinds of wonders in the body, including the reduction of triglycerides. When your annual blood work shows lower triglycerides, this indicates that your blood sugar is probably within a healthy range and you're in an anti-aging mode.
- You'll be keeping your blood sugar at a healthy level with this plan, naturally and efficiently. The foods you'll be emphasizing are rich in soluble fiber; I'm talking about fruits, veggies, and certain grains like oatmeal and barley. Soluble fiber thickens digested food so sugar gets absorbed more slowly, over a longer time, thus avoiding sugar spikes. Adding protein-rich foods to meals and snacks also aids in keeping your blood sugar stable. Some protein is converted into sugar by the liver and then pumped out slowly into the bloodstream, just about the time when the sugar from fruits and vegetables is declining. The healthy fats you'll be eating slow down digestion and absorption even more, keeping you feeling full longer.

Voilà! This plan is a natural solution that prevents roller-coaster rides of blood sugar and kicks age-promoting added sugar out of your life.

Finding Sugars

To see if a food contains any sort of added sugar, look for these on the ingredient label. Even better, skip processed foods altogether!

Agave nectar	Golden sugar
Barley malt	Golden syrup
Beet sugar	Granulated sugar
Blackstrap molasses	Grape juice concentrate
Brown sugar	Grape sugar
Cane crystals	High-fructose corn syrup
Cane sugar	Honey
Caramel	Invert sugar
Confectioner's sugar	Lactose
Corn sweetener	Malt syrup
Corn syrup	Maltodextrin
Corn syrup solids	Maltose
Crystalline fructose	Maple syrup
Date sugar	Molasses
Dextrin	Organic raw sugar
Dextrose	Powdered sugar
Evaporated cane juice	Raw sugar
Fructose	Rice syrup
Fruit juice	Sorghum syrup
Fruit juice concentrate	Sucrose
Galactose	Sugar
Glucose	Table sugar
Glucose solids	Turbinado sugar

CHAPTER 6

Fire Big Food and Big Pharma

Aging is like skiing downhill. Once you start, it's hard to stop—especially if you've been given a push by Big Food and Big Pharma. By Big Food, I mean large commercial entities or conglomerates that dominate the production of food and beverages worldwide. One of their main goals is to produce food more cheaply for maximum profit—that often means nutrient-empty processed food—and to get you to buy lots of it. Big Pharma refers to the large drug companies that are selling drugs, in many cases, for diseases that can be prevented by lifestyle changes—drugs that can actually accelerate the aging process.

There are many ways to stop the slide, and I've talked about them—plant foods, flavonoids, less added sugar, and probiotics. These measures can give you a healthy body—one that resists aging. That said, I want to talk to you about two more actions that will further put the brakes on aging. First, stop eating highly processed foods; and second, look to food, rather than pills, as medicine that's good for what ails you.

Big Food: If You Are What You Eat, How Do You Like Being Processed?

In very simple terms, there are only two categories of food: whole foods and processed foods. Whole foods are those that haven't been tampered with, in the lab or the manufacturing plant. They contain all their original nutrients and come straight from nature: especially whole fruits and vegetables and basically the core foods of the DASH Diet Younger You plan.

By definition, a processed food has been altered from its natural state. Certain foods have always been processed, initially for good reason. Cooking and preservation methods are types of processing; they have helped make food safer and more digestible. And minimally processed foods, which I recommend, include reduced fat dairy, fermented foods, and frozen fruits and vegetables (without any additives). Today, though, "processed" normally refers to foods that are packaged in boxes, cans, or bags—and have been adulterated with trans fats, saturated fats, large amounts of sodium and sugar, and other additives. It's easy to tell whether a food is processed. Just look at the ingredient list. The longer the list, the more processed a food is likely to be. Unfortunately, most people are still clinging to a diet of mostly processed foods. In fact, it has been reported that 90 percent of all food consumed in the United States today is processed. Fraught with problems, processed food:

- Is often depleted of the normal nutritional value of whole food. No wonder we are so malnourished as a society!
- Contains additives such as added sugars, bad fats, and potentially dangerous substitutes like preservatives and colorings.
- Is packaged in paper impregnated with potentially hazardous fluorochemicals (chemically similar to those used to make

nonstick pans, and who wants to be nonstick from the inside out?) or plastics impregnated with BPA (bisphenol A), plasticizers, or phthalates.

- Is full of pro-aging ingredients: trans fats, which promote inflammation and interfere with your ability to fight aging; and genetically modified organisms (GMOs), which can promote weight gain and permanently alter the composition and function of the microbiota in your gut. Since they are still relatively new, GMOs may also have unknown long-term effects.

- Shortens telomeres. Using data from 840 adults from the Multi-Ethnic Study of U.S. Atherosclerosis, researchers found strong associations between diet and telomere length. Reporting in the *American Journal of Clinical Nutrition* in 2008, they noted that eating a lot of processed meats like bacon, sausage, luncheon meats, and ham could shorten your telomeres.

- Encourages obesity, a pro-aging condition. Not only does obesity promote life-threatening illnesses and inflammation, it also promotes a life-shortening reality: It shortens telomeres. But don't panic if you're not happy with the number on the scale: Losing weight can restore the length of telomeres, and you can definitely drop pounds on this plan.

These alarming problems have largely to do with the rise of Big Food. Like many other food experts, I know that Big Food tries to make processed food irresistible to consumers. They do this by carefully lacing food with precise, calculated ratios of sugar, fat, and salt designed to stimulate the brain so we literally get addicted to the food and can't resist it. There's no question: We're being processed. Our taste buds are being co-opted, and our food preferences are being programmed. Many experts compare the addictive nature and danger of processed foods to the addictive nature and danger of tobacco and cigarettes. Both the tobacco companies and Big Food are brilliant at marketing their products to consumers so they can't resist them and get hooked.

I'm not immune to this, either! I love potato chips and Snickers and could eat them all day long. But then I would be immense, I would probably have high blood pressure and be diabetic, and I would look awful. So, I don't eat that way. Some people have told me that their cravings for such foods mean their body is telling them what they need, so they don't feel they should stop eating junk foods. But do you ever hear people say they crave broccoli, which is actually important? When I hear people insist that they can't give up their favorite junk foods, I share with them my extreme example, to illustrate the problem with thinking that their body "knows" what to eat. We need to change. If we want different results, we have to take different actions. Today, we have epidemics of obesity, diabetes, and other chronic diseases—driven by ever-increasing calories, added sugar, salt, artery-clogging fats, and processed starch—created by Big Food. Then along comes Big Pharma to treat us.

It's all just part of the...process.

Are we supposed to be okay with this?

No, we can free ourselves of The Process—with the DASH Diet Younger You plan.

Big Food and Big Farm

Another aspect of Big Food is the factory farm (often called Big Farm), where livestock are pumped full of antibiotics and hormones so that they fatten up and produce more meat and milk faster. It's well known that animals on factory farms are often kept in conditions that are less than humane. They may be confined to tiny areas, not large enough to move or lie down in. They may be fed genetically modified (GMO) grains. All of these practices have helped produce abundant supplies of foods at low cost. However, they have also led to more frequent contamination of foods with antibiotic-resistant organisms and may be introducing unneeded hormones that could be making us fatter, too.

Our agricultural policies led to high production of corn and wheat—and in turn led to nutritional policies that placed an emphasis on grains as the foundation of our diets. Those grains are mostly processed. In the process of turning whole wheat into white flour, manufacturers strip away the bran (the outside covering) and the germ (not a microorganism germ, but the part of the seed that grows into the new plant). The wheat flour then lacks vital nutrients like vitamins, minerals, and fiber but is "enriched" by adding a few nutrients—but not the same ones that were removed. There are now a lot of starchy packaged foods in the grocery stores, with tantalizing labels like "enriched" duping people into thinking these foods are healthy. But they aren't as healthy as the natural whole foods—foods that don't need to be enriched. Nor are they any lower in calories. And most of us are not physically active enough to burn off all those calories from the large amounts of grain that too many of us have been consuming.

Corn, in particular, is used to make corn syrup, cornstarch, grits, cornmeal, high-fructose corn syrup (HFCS), cereals, and more. Most U.S.-grown corn actually gets used for industrial products, rather than for food. However, we do end up with a lot of corn-derived products in our foods. And although we hear a lot these days about wheat and gluten sensitivity, many people are unaware that corn is also a common allergen. I personally have a very mild corn allergy, which makes my face puffy and aggravates my sinuses. Puffiness and other symptoms brought on by hidden mild food allergies or intolerances make us feel and look old, unless we stop eating the offending food. Since these food ingredients are so pervasive in processed foods, it can be difficult to get to the root cause of our symptoms unless we focus on unprocessed, whole foods.

Big Food and Big Farm are also involved in spreading the use of genetically modified crops. GMO plants are often created by introducing a gene from one species into the DNA of a completely different species—like splicing fish genes into tomato chromosomes, a totally unnatural process. The only upside of genetic engineering is that it does allow grains to be produced with less pesticides, which can be a benefit. Still, I'd prefer to not eat Frankenfoods!

Grains, including GMO grains such as corn, are fed to beef cattle—another unfortunate Big Farm practice, since grain-fed beef may not have the same nutritional properties as grass-fed beef. Plus, grass-fed beef is leaner and more flavorful, though sometimes less tender, than grain-fed beef. Grass-fed beef is richer in many important vitamins and minerals and high in certain healthy fats, including the body-protective omega-3 fats.

A final point here: Beef cattle are also pumped up with hormones, such as estrogen, to make them fatter more quickly. This practice is scary: We may be ingesting those hormones when we eat the beef, and those hormones can possibly affect our weight and increase the risk for some cancers. They fatten the animal, but they may also fatten us. Fortunately, chicken and pork are not raised with added hormones, which are banned under federal law. To avoid hormone- and antibiotic-treated livestock, look for products labeled "hormone-free" and "antibiotic-free."

Big Pharma: Are You Pilling Yourself?

First, my disclaimer. In no way would I ever recommend that you discontinue any medication your physician has prescribed.

But if you're taking medicine, some of the concepts here might help you take less of that medication or ease off it altogether—of course, only with your doctor's guidance.

And if you are among those people who aren't taking any meds, there are many steps you can take nutritionally to help avoid them in the future.

For perspective, many commonly prescribed medications may actually trigger some of the diseases of aging, such as heart disease and diabetes, and can make you feel and look older.

Hypertension Medication

Let's start with blood pressure medications, which are used to treat heart conditions. Some blood pressure medications, for example, cause women to lose hair, particularly on the crown of their head. Some people will develop a chronic cough. And it is well known that some blood pressure meds interfere with sexual prowess. But few people know that diuretics can increase the risk of developing type 2 diabetes, within one year. What's more, an increasing number of people are being put on these meds when they may not really need them. There are two reasons for this. For people with stage 1 hypertension, the DASH diet has been proven to reverse hypertension in fourteen days, performing as well as the first-line medications. But many physicians think their patients won't really make changes in their eating habits and so don't even recommend it. And several years ago, a new condition called prehypertension was labeled by the medical establishment. This new label was based on research indicating that blood pressure higher than 115 over 70 was already starting to cause damage to arteries and blood vessels. Physicians recommended reversing prehypertension—a great goal, but some wanted to do it with medication.

Is that the best course of action? I don't think so. Many people can reverse prehypertension with diet alone. The DASH diet does this, and literally makes your blood vessels younger from the inside out. Adding exercise helps, too. You can reverse prehypertension by lifestyle changes alone.

Even better, following the DASH diet also reduces your risk of heart attack, stroke, and heart failure (which is a direct consequence of high blood pressure, particularly if uncontrolled, hindering the heart from pumping as strongly). This is an important issue to men and women, but my women readers should really take note.

Women: After you have a heart attack, you may not fully recover, and in fact, a majority do not. Also, you're more likely to have a stroke than are men. Strokes can be debilitating, and it can take years, if ever, to regain functional abilities.

Heart attacks and strokes can age you tremendously. A large part of looking younger is related to feeling younger. If you *feel* energetic, you will be more motivated to *stay* young and vital. You're more likely to dress younger, keep your hair and makeup up to date, and stay current with fashion. When you feel older or suffer from debilitating diseases, you may lose your will to maintain a high quality of life.

I DASHed Aging!

An interesting thing happened to me after I started the DASH Diet Younger You plan. Even though I lost eight pounds the first two weeks, I wasn't feeling 100 percent. It turned out that the diet naturally lowered my blood pressure, and since I was taking hypertension meds, my blood pressure got too low. I knew DASH could lower blood pressure, but I didn't know it could happen so fast. After seeing these results, my doctor took me off the medication. All I can say is: Amazing!

—*Lucy E.*

Diabetes Drugs

If you're diagnosed with prediabetes or full-blown diabetes, you'll generally be prescribed medications as a first line of defense. Be careful here: Diabetes medications can actually speed the progression of the disease. That's bad, because diabetes is already an aging disease. Adding in the prescription drugs is like tossing an accelerant onto a fire. The result: even faster aging.

A common diabetes medication is a class of drugs known as sulfonylureas. They help your body produce more insulin, but in doing so, they make the insulin-secreting cells in the pancreas wear out faster.

Another commonly prescribed med is metformin. It helps your body respond better to insulin but can produce diarrhea so severe that you might even become homebound, concerned that you will have a severe attack when or where you can't properly deal with it. Even worse, the diarrhea reduces your absorption of key nutrients, especially minerals, that are necessary for proper insulin function.

And if you need to go on insulin with type 2 diabetes, you'll most surely gain a significant amount of weight. Here's why: You'll be losing less sugar in your urine, and that retained sugar will be converted into body fat. The insulin you're taking can increase hunger and cause more fat to be deposited around your belly. None of these side effects will make you feel any younger or healthier. (Note that taking insulin for type 1 diabetes is unavoidable because the body doesn't make insulin at all.)

Fortunately, type 2 diabetes and prediabetes respond exceptionally well to changes in diet, exercise, and lifestyle. Exercise is more effective at treating and reversing type 2 diabetes than any medication ever developed. The reason is that it makes muscle cells more receptive to insulin, and then you start processing blood sugar normally.

When you control diabetes with lifestyle changes, you'll be able to better resist aging, because you've resisted diabetes-produced aging and you've opted not to take age-promoting diabetes drugs. But many people prefer the ease of taking diabetes medication, unaware of the consequences.

I can't tell you how many times I've had clients with diabetes who were much younger than I but looked and physically *were* ten to twenty years older. It was always shocking to me to hear them say that they believed aging so quickly was unavoidable. I personally do not expect to age. I plan to stay young looking, feeling, and acting, by avoiding my family history of diabetes through diet and exercise.

The DASH Diet Younger You plan is the perfect dietary way to control diabetes. It gets you off refined starchy and added-sugar foods immediately, and this reduces the demand on your pancreas to produce insulin. It reduces your intake of trans fats and saturated fats in order to reduce inflammation and oxidative stress, both of which can hasten diabetes development. And exercise helps burn off blood sugar and helps you respond better to insulin, so your pancreas doesn't have to overproduce it, preserving your ability to make insulin.

3 Meds That Affect You in Bed

Taking drugs and suffering from a lack of libido? It's no wonder, since a slew of prescription meds can dampen your sex life. Here's a look at three offenders:

Blood Pressure Drugs. If you're a guy with high blood pressure, this condition could affect your erectile function. Taking drugs for high blood pressure may worsen the problem, unfortunately. Follow the DASH Diet Younger You plan and monitor your blood pressure. You may be able to get off the medication and resume a normal, active sex life.

Antidepressants. The mood elevators might lift your mood, but they suppress your libido, delay ejaculation, and make it difficult to reach orgasm. I'm confident that if you follow the DASH Diet Younger You plan, you'll be able to chase the blues away naturally, without drugs—and thus get rid of these sexual side effects. Also, regular exercise, along with the right diet, has been shown to help with symptoms of depression, high blood pressure, and impotence.

Heartburn Drugs. Studies have found that these drugs, used to reduce stomach acid and treat acid reflux, may cause erectile dysfunction. I've had clients who were able to get off these drugs after being on the DASH diet, with its abundance of probiotics and prebiotics. Plus, it cuts out fatty and fried foods, both known to trigger heartburn. A nutritional fix like DASH is worth a try to revive your sex life. And heartburn meds can also lead to anemia, because they reduce absorption of iron and vitamin B12.

Bone-Strengthening Drugs

Another area where prescription drugs can age us is in bone health. As we age, both men and women progressively lose calcium from our bones. This problem is more pronounced in postmenopausal women. You can find out if you're losing calcium by having a bone density test, a simple type of X-ray that determines the concentration of calcium in your bones, usually at the hip and spine.

If you've lost a significant but not extreme amount of calcium, your doctor may diagnose a condition called osteopenia. There is a lot of debate as to whether it is a disease or just a natural part of aging, just as skin wrinkles are not a disease. Nonetheless, physicians these days want to treat it with medications to prevent the condition from getting worse: female hormones or other prescription meds to arrest the process and maintain bone strength. The problem with bone medications is that they actually increase the number of "old bone cells" in your body, rather than rejuvenating your bones by creating young cells. And the hormones increase risk of stroke and heart attacks.

Before turning to drugs, however, you can avoid further bone loss with lifestyle measures: a calcium-rich diet (yogurt, low-fat dairy foods, and green leafy vegetables), regular strength-training and cardio exercises, ample intake of calcium and vitamin D, no smoking, and alcohol consumption limited to no more than two drinks a day. For years, bone loss was treated with calcium supplements, too. Now we know that there is almost no benefit from these supplements, and, in fact, they may increase your risk for plaque buildup in your arteries.

Unchecked, osteopenia can lead to osteoporosis, a very crippling bone disease. It, too, can be halted with lifestyle changes and medication. But the key is not to let osteopenia progress to osteoporosis.

Other Medication Issues

A lot of people are prescribed "water pills" (thiazides) for various conditions, from simple bloating to high blood pressure to heart conditions. Unfortunately, these meds can increase the risk of developing diabetes within one year of use.

Similarly, many people take statins, prescribed to normalize cholesterol, but these, too, increase the risk of developing diabetes, especially if you're female. Statins can also cause muscle weakness, heartburn, forgetfulness, and is associated with increased risk for age-related macular degeneration, along with other signs of aging.

Even more problematic, many people think that if they're taking pills for their health conditions, they don't need to worry about food choices any longer. And nothing could be further from the truth.

Pills treat symptoms; they don't make you healthier. For example, taking medication may help lower your cholesterol, but it doesn't do anything to extend your longevity. Eating healthier has been proven to be associated with a longer life span.

My advice here is to be medically savvy. Know the side effects of meds you're prescribed. Find out what lifestyle measures you can take before taking medications. Be skeptical when you see TV commercials touting prescription drugs. They're selling the underlying message that our lifestyles can be improved with drugs. Not true. I always find it ironic that these commercials show enticing scenes of people enjoying life because of the drug, while the soothing narration lists the potentially dangerous side effects of that drug! Drugs may artificially lower numbers that are markers of disease, like cholesterol, blood sugar, or blood pressure, but they may not address the cause of the problem, creating perpetual drug dependency.

The only way you can make your body truly healthier and younger is to choose to eat a variety of real, mostly plant-based foods and to be physically active. In other words, to follow the DASH Diet Younger You program.

The concept is not new. In ancient times, Hippocrates gave similar wise advice: "Let your food be your medicine."

Now we know that Hippocrates was a true visionary.

DASH Wrinkles: Avoid Pollutants

We're exposed to pollutants in the environment every day, from the food we eat to the air we breathe. Fortunately, our skin is a major protective barrier between our bodies and pollutants, which include UV rays from the sun, cigarette smoke, fuel exhaust and soot, air pollution, and others. These pollutants

(continued)

promote oxid-aging and the production of free radicals that can damage skin cells and accelerate aging in general.

Here's how you can protect your skin against these threats—and prevent or minimize wrinkles:

- Eat more organic fruits and vegetables; they contain fewer toxic pesticides and are high in antioxidants that fight oxid-aging.

- Stay away from cigarette smoke. It will age you and the people around you. You won't get the youthful look you want if you continue smoking or exposing yourself to secondhand smoke.

- Hydrate your skin. Drink pure water throughout the day, six to eight glasses (unless your physician has prescribed a lower intake). Water eliminates toxins and pollutants from your system, so it's a wonderful flushing and cleansing agent for your body.

Supplements: When Big Food Meets Big Pharma

In recent years, the vitamin, supplement, and herbal remedy companies have been invaded by the major pharmaceutical groups (Big Pharma), with drug companies purchasing supplement companies—which puts supplements at the intersection of Big Food and Big Pharma. The major reason for the invasion is that pipelines of new drug products are running dry and Big Pharma needs other sources of revenue. With Big Pharma adding dietary supplements to its lines, what assurances do we as consumers have about exactly what we're getting, and about the safety of the products we buy?

Short answer: Not many. Unlike the regulation of food or pharmaceuticals, U.S. law does not require supplement manufacturers to get FDA approval for their products. The manufacturers themselves are responsible for ensuring that their products are safe, and they do not have to report any testing results to the FDA. This is a little (or a lot) looser assurance than I personally am comfortable with. There is a wide range of herbs that have potential health and rejuvenation benefits. But I prefer to cook with these herbs, rather than to have someone else extract some component of them and assure me that this processed fraction is what I need.

Many supplement manufacturers pull apart foods or herbs and sell their extracted components without thinking about what they might be losing. We've learned a lot about all the phytonutrients in plant-based foods, but research has always shown that eating the complete foods is what really makes us healthy. Plants contain so many healthful components, and it appears to be the combination of all the nutrients that provides the benefits. For example, raspberries aren't just about anti-aging anthocyanins; they are also rich in fiber and contain quercetin and gallic acid, which help prevent heart disease. We won't get the full benefit from having an anthocyanin supplement. Even more troubling, in many supplements (even if you think you are taking natural herbs), you may find that there are other additives, and in some cases, regulators have seen that the supplement doesn't even contain the herb listed on the label. Although deconstructed foods are a fad, when it comes to health, it is better not to deconstruct the food or the herbs and spices.

Then there is the scary research showing that some supplements do not give the benefits once expected, or in some cases do more harm than good. We discussed some of this research in Chapter 2 (see the section titled "Can't I Just Pop Antioxidant Supplements?"). Take vitamin E, for example. Back in 1999, Italian researchers reported in the journal *Lancet* that vitamin E—once hailed as heart-healthy—showed no effect in a study of more than 11,000 heart attack survivors. Since then, even more research has turned up the same findings.

Also, a recent study looked into whether vitamin E and selenium supplements could prevent prostate cancer. Lo and behold, the researchers stopped the study abruptly after discovering that the people on vitamin E showed an increased risk of prostate cancer!

What do we make of all this? As you can probably tell by now, I'm no fan of dietary supplements. I believe we are designed to absorb all necessary nutrients from a healthy diet, and so supplementing intake levels beyond this is unwise. My advice is simple: Eat a wide variety of fresh, whole foods, mostly plants, in moderation, and exercise regularly.

The Perils of Packaging

The food we buy often comes in packages made with BPA (bisphenol A), an additive that can age us. Another such additive is DEHP (diethylhexyl phthalate), though BPA is the more notorious.

BPA is used in many types of food packaging. The major concern is that in high concentrations, it can have hormone-like properties, which may be linked to developmental and fertility problems, weight gain, as well as cancers, heart disease, and brain disorders.

In general, plastics that are marked with Resin Identification Codes 1, 2, 4, 5, and 6, as shown below this paragraph, are very unlikely to contain BPA. Most cans used as food packaging in the United States are lined with plastics containing BPA. There is controversy about whether BPA is safe in food packaging, with no reliable studies showing harm, but continuing caution about the possibility of endocrine disruption. Scientific evidence does not show that there is any effect in humans at the very low dosages used in food packaging. But it should be noted that BPA is found in the tissues of the vast majority of Americans. If you are trying to avoid additives, skipping the packaging that contains BPA may be something to consider.

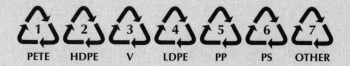

To avoid BPA:

- Eat less canned food. Instead, choose frozen or fresh fruits and vegetables—always a better choice, anyway.

- If you use containers that you suspect are made of BPA, don't put them in your microwave to heat up food or liquids. The heat causes BPA to leach from the container into the food.

- If you drink bottled water, consider switching from a BPA-containing plastic bottle to one made of stainless steel.

Is Organic the Answer for Anti-Aging?

Organic foods have become big business, too. You can find many large chains of "whole foods" grocers selling organic foods and even organic sections in your regular supermarket.

The chief benefit of eating organic foods is that they lower your body's "toxic burden." Often unbeknownst to us, we're exposed to toxins in the environment every day—in our food, in the air, all around us. Among these toxins are pesticides, typically sprayed on fruits and vegetables to protect them from insects. Pesticides can enter our bodies and cause slow, subtle damage. Our bodies will store pesticides in fat tissue, and the more fat you have, the more of these toxins you will store.

It is possible to reduce exposure to pesticides by purchasing organic foods. They are not sprayed with pesticides. Nor is organic livestock treated with hormones or antibiotics. Choosing organic foods is another helpful step you can take toward anti-aging and good health.

But organic foods are not only lower in toxins, they're also higher in beneficial antioxidants and therefore prevent oxid-aging. In fact, organic foods have more antioxidants than conventionally grown foods; research backs up this fact.

To reduce your toxic burden:

- Definitely look for produce that is grown organically, if it fits into your budget.
- Purchase foods from farmers' markets—where you may find many participating farmers who raise food organically.
- Subscribe to a community-supported agricultural program (CSA), from which you can receive boxes of organically grown produce weekly or every few weeks. A CSA service can introduce you to new vegetables.
- Grow your own, either in your yard, at a community garden, or if space is a problem, in pots. Growing my own is my favorite solution. The taste of fresh produce is superior to any you can buy, and the vitamins have full potency, with none of the loss that happens while they are sitting on the shelves in the stores. And I know for sure that no artificial pesticides were used on my produce!
- Purchase grass-fed beef. Although it can be more expensive than conventionally raised beef, it is free of hormones and

antibiotics. If you can find local farmers who grow grass-fed, you can order a side or a quarter of beef to cut the cost down to what you would pay for regular beef. You'll need a freezer to store it, but it will certainly make it easy to pull out what you need, without having to go to the store. You could also try buying the quarter or side of beef with some friends, if you don't want to store too much. You'll learn to try new cuts of beef, and also how to avoid overcooking steaks and burgers, since lean beef (and in fact any lean meat) can get tough if overcooked.

- Beware of labels that say "natural." Foods that say "natural" on the package probably aren't. This is a hot issue right now, since the word "natural" isn't regulated. Many packaged vegetarian foods and meat substitutes made with soy, for example, are highly processed. My first job after college was in research for a major soybean processor. I have seen the processing up close. Instead of buying processed vegetarian foods, make your own. I have included lots of vegetarian recipes in this book that will help you. My mantra is: If the package has to say it's natural, it probably isn't!

- Watch out for gluten-free foods. Many packaged gluten-free foods are based on highly processed flours. Fortunately, with the DASH Diet Younger You plan, you don't need to be overly concerned with how to live gluten-free without processed foods, since you'll be eating foods that are mostly gluten-free anyway.

DASH Big Food and Big Pharma

As you follow the DASH Diet Younger You plan, you'll automatically be excluding refined, highly processed foods from your diet and all the additives needed to stabilize them. Also, you'll rely less on Big Pharma by getting all the healthy protective benefits of DASH, most notably its blood-pressure-lowering and cholesterol-lowering effects.

One of the first things my clients say after just a few days on this plan is that they feel so much better and cleaner. This is the body eliminating toxins and getting younger.

PART II

Put Old on Hold

CHAPTER 7

Younger You Meal Plans

Here is where I put the previously discussed five strategies into action; in other words, here's how your diet looks when you incorporate these breakthrough strategies. This includes menus with ideas for a variety of meals and snacks for vegetarians, and menus for those who include poultry, fish, and meat in their diet.

This plan provides plenty of options to suit your tastes. And feel free to mix and match meals, or to make substitutions of foods with others that have similar nutritional properties. The plan is packed with fourteen days of completely meatless meal options, plus fourteen days of meals with fish, poultry, and even a few dishes for the beef lovers. Some of the meals with chicken also have tofu substitutes or you can substitute a different bean dish from the recipe chapter. You can be as meatless as you want to be. People want to follow the DASH diet because it is so healthy, and now you can take it to the next level while it makes you younger!

Protein-Rich Foods

The DASH Diet Younger You program is incredibly simple to follow. The foods you'll be eating include a variety of fruits and vegetables and are mostly plant-based. Even though I don't emphasize lots of meat on the DASH program, the plan still provides your body with all the protein it needs for strong muscles and good health. Whether from vegetarian sources or animal sources, here's a guide to meeting the protein requirements of this plan in the healthiest way.

Whether you are vegetarian or are simply trying to eat less meat, it is easy for you to choose healthy plant-based proteins. I am not a big fan of the heavily processed, packaged "fake" meat substitutes, but there are lots of naturally high-protein vegetarian foods, like beans, to choose from. Beans will always be good for you. They are high in fiber, good sources of minerals and protein, and most are very low-fat. The DASH Diet Younger You program has many meals and recipes based on beans, so you will find lots of ideas. New to beans? Go slowly when adding them to your diet.

When choosing fish, opt for wild fish rather than farm-raised. It can be difficult to tell what you are getting at restaurants, but a clue is the width of the fat bands. The wider the bands, the more likely that the fish was farmed. You want wild, because it will be the richest in the omega-3 fats that are so healthy and good for your heart. Otherwise, what's the point? All tuna will be wild, and your best choices are albacore and bluefin tuna, for the maximum amount of omega-3s. Not everyone is a fan of herring, sardines, and anchovies, but they are also excellent sources of omega-3s.

With chicken and turkey, you don't have to worry about hormones, but you may want to buy and eat humanely raised and organic poultry. You can now find these at most grocery stores, at organic food stores, and often from local farmers' markets. The same goes for eggs. If you can get locally raised eggs, go for it! And if you are lucky enough to have the space, interest, and local zoning allowances to raise your own, I am envious of you. Or perhaps you have friends or neighbors who are raising chickens and may be willing to share some of those eggs. I usually buy vegetarian-fed, cage-free eggs, which I find taste better, as well as being lower in cholesterol.

When shopping for beef, look for organically raised beef, or for a slightly higher price, grass-fed beef. Cows are natural grass eaters, so grass-fed cows are eating a healthier and more natural diet, making their meat more nutritious for you. The grass-fed beef will be higher in some important fats, such as omega-3s and conjugated linoleic acid (CLA), which improve the beef's nutritional profile. Grass-fed beef will be leaner, so be careful not to overcook, or it will become dry. If you have local farmers raising grass-fed beef, partner with your neighbors to buy a half or a quarter of a cow, so that you don't have to stock as much in your freezer.

With dairy, you want to choose mostly low-fat and nonfat dairy. Some people are anti–reduced-fat dairy. However, there is nothing unnatural about skimming off the butterfat; this has been done throughout recorded history, long before the dairy industry came to be. In fact, the real challenge is getting the fat to stay in the milk, which is why milk is homogenized. Most reduced-fat cheeses have no extra additives; they just use reduced-fat milk as the starting ingredient. They may have a preservative to inhibit mold development, but if you are, like me, allergic to mold, you will appreciate that. If you are occasionally having fabulous gourmet cheeses that aren't low-fat, enjoy! But keep the rest of the meal centered on vegetables and fruits, to avoid overdoing saturated fats. Yogurt is a fabulous source of "good bacteria" for your gut. I recommend either low-fat or nonfat. I've included a recipe with various suggestions to help you add flavor to plain yogurt (without adding artificial sweeteners), in Chapter 8. In general, I discourage Greek yogurt (yes, I know it is so creamy and is higher in protein), because much of the potassium and calcium is lost during the filtration process, and these are the key minerals that you need for the DASH diet to work. You also lose much of the whey protein, which is a real powerhouse for building and maintaining muscle. I apologize in advance if you love Greek yogurt. Keep it as a treat, rather than a regular dairy food.

Fruits, Vegetables, and Grains

Fruits and vegetables are, of course, high in all those desirable antioxidants, including the powerful flavonoids. With fruits and vegetables that have thick skins and need to be peeled before eating, you can get away without choosing organically grown. But if the produce doesn't get peeled, you will definitely have a huge reduction in pesticides if you buy organic or grow your own. With berries, it is especially beneficial to choose organic, because it is so hard to fully wash off residual pesticides. Frozen produce is as good as fresh. This is one of those cases where minimally processing (blanching and freezing) preserves the nutritional profile of the foods, and frozen produce can actually be healthier than unprocessed produce that has been sitting in bins in the store for a long time. If you want to avoid canned foods, you can find boxed ("canned" without the can) tomatoes in many supermarkets. If you have an Italian or Mediterranean market in your neighborhood, check it out, since they may have more choices of "uncanned" tomato products.

Packaged foods based on grains, like boxed cereals, crackers, and cereal bars, are most likely to be processed. Oatmeal, homemade granola, and 100 percent whole grain or bran cereals are the least likely of the cereals to be processed. Most breads are highly processed. I choose a light whole wheat bread, to keep the calories under control. Most light breads either are very thinly sliced, or are more "airy" as a way of cutting the calories. You can also choose breads with wheat berries (much of which passes through your body, undigested) or sprouted grain breads. If you want to minimize additives, you can make your own, or just limit the amount you consume. Pasta can also be very low in additives, and whole grain is best. You can also find noodles made with beans in Asian markets, or in the Asian food aisle in a regular grocery store. If you have any trouble finding these foods in your local stores, you can find almost everything available online, so you can experiment even if you live in a remote region or just a place with a poor selection of grocery stores.

To show you a variety of ideas on how to put together the DASH Diet Younger You plan meals, I have included fourteen days of vegetarian meals, seven days of meals for fish and poultry lovers, and seven days of meals that include some red meat. You can mix or match all of the meals and snacks. Choose the ones you love and use them as models for continuing variations based on your own tastes. You do, however, want to come pretty close to following the DASH diet eating pattern on most days—read on for details.

Anti-Aging Beverages vs. Aging Beverages

The cleanest flavored beverage is water with slices of fresh fruit or vegetables. My favorites include lemon, orange, grapefruit, and cucumber slices. You can also try adding chunks of watermelon, honeydew, or cantaloupe. Another simple way to add flavor with minimal calories is to freeze fresh lemon, orange, or grapefruit juice in an ice tray. Then add a few of the citrus ice cubes to your water for a flavorful, refreshing drink.

Coffee and tea without added sugar are very healthy. We used to think caffeine was bad for you, but now we have seen that there are many benefits to consuming caffeine. Caffeine

(continued)

improves athletic performance, in addition to being well known for improving alertness. Both black and green teas are full of antioxidants. Coffee is very rich in potassium, which is associated with reducing fluid retention and improving blood pressure. People who are regular heavy coffee drinkers are less likely to develop type 2 diabetes. It used to be thought that caffeinated beverages were dehydrating; however, the net benefit is overwhelmingly for hydration. The problem with caffeinated beverages comes mostly from additives such as sugars and cream.

Red wine, as I noted earlier, is rich in antioxidants. Some studies have suggested that it helps reduce blood cholesterol after a rich, meaty meal. And people who drink alcohol moderately have a lower risk of dying than those who do not drink at all and those who are heavy drinkers.

That said, I am anti-smoothies, protein shakes, and juicing. I prefer to have people eating food, as opposed to drinking their calories. Four fluid ounces of juice each day is fine, but most people consume much more than this. Blenders either remove fiber or pulverize it, making it almost worthless. Then the sugar just surges into your bloodstream. We love whole fruits and veggies precisely because they are bulky and filling and take longer to eat. Have lots of fruits and veggies, but please eat them, don't drink them.

Most people need the equivalent of eight to ten glasses of fluid each day. This includes fruits, veggies, milk, and yogurt, because they are mostly water. And even meat, fish, and poultry contribute lots of water. Most people will find this very easy to accomplish, especially with our focus on fresh, whole foods. But absolutely, do feel free to drink lots of water. With the increased fiber in the DASH Diet Younger You plan, it will help promote digestive health.

The DASH Eating Plan

So what should you eat every day, and how much of it? Here's a helpful chart that outlines foods to emphasize and foods to limit, with clear guidelines so that you know what to put on your plate at every meal. The meal plans in this chapter have already done the math and planning for you. I have tried to make this plan fun by including wine. If you don't imbibe, substitute another serving of fruit.

The DASH Diet
Younger You Recommended Daily Servings

Nonstarchy vegetables	Unlimited, at least 4 servings, and preferably 5 or more
Starchy vegetables	Count as a vegetable serving, but limit to no more than 1–2 per week, especially if trying to lose weight
Fruit	3–5 servings
Dairy	At least 2–3 servings
Nuts, seeds	1–2 servings
Lean meat, fish, poultry, eggs, beans	5–8 ounces of meat fish, poultry, eggs, or a little more for larger men. One egg or 2 egg whites is the equivalent of 1 ounce of meat. ½ cup beans equals the calories of 3 ounces of meat but has the protein of 1 ounce.
Fats	1–3 servings
Whole grains	2–3 servings
Refined grains, sweets	Rarely, 2–3 times per week, maximum

Serving Sizes for the DASH Diet Younger You

All serving sizes are as consumed. For example, rice and oatmeal servings are the cooked serving sizes. Meat serving sizes are also cooked portions, and generally about 25 percent of the weight is lost during cooking, so that four ounces of uncooked meat yields three ounces of cooked meat. To evaluate foods that are not on this list or that may be ambiguous, I have included representative calories for these serving sizes. These serving sizes are largely consistent with the diabetic exchange list, except for nuts.

Grains, starches (80 calories per serving)

1 slice of bread
½ English muffin or bun
¼ bagel
1 ounce dry cereal, ½ cup cooked cereal, pasta, corn, rice, or
    starchy vegetables, including potatoes and winter squash

Fruits (60 calories per serving)

4 ounces fruit by weight
4 fluid ounces juice
1 small piece of fruit
½ cup canned, frozen fruit
¼ cup dried fruit

Vegetables (25–30 calories for nonstarchy, 80 calories for starchy)

½ cup cooked or raw vegetables
1 cup leafy raw vegetables
4 fluid ounces vegetable juice

Dairy (90–100 calories per serving)

8 fluid ounces (1 cup) milk, yogurt

1 ounce cheese

½ cup cottage cheese

Meats, fish, poultry (140–200 calories per serving)

3 ounces, cooked

Eggs (80 calories)

1 egg

2 egg whites

Beans (160 calories per serving)

½ cup cooked beans, lentils, or peas

Nuts (180 calories per serving)

¼ cup or 1 ounce nuts

2 tablespoons or 1 ounce seeds

2 tablespoons peanut butter

Fats and oils (35–40 calories per serving)

1 teaspoon butter

1 teaspoon vegetable oil

1 slice avocado

Beverages

Wine: 3½ fluid ounces has 90 calories; 5 fluid ounces has
    125 calories

Substitution Foods If You Have Allergies

The most common allergies and intolerances include wheat, fish and/or shellfish, peanuts and tree nuts, soy, eggs, and dairy. And I will add two of my own, mold and corn.

More and more people are either being diagnosed with Crohn's disease or have discovered that they have some kind of wheat sensitivity. With the DASH Diet Younger You program, this is so easy to accommodate. You do not need to eat any wheat products. And when you are eating fresh, whole, unprocessed (or minimally processed) foods, you won't have as much risk of consuming hidden ingredients that introduce gluten into your meals. The heart of this diet plan is automatically gluten-free. When I recommend whole wheat breads or cereals, use gluten-free substitutes if you are avoiding gluten.

If you are allergic to soy products, this plan will make it easy to stay on track, again, because the fresh, whole foods do not have the hidden ingredients that can sneak up on you in processed foods.

If you have allergies to fish, shellfish, peanuts, and tree nuts, your allergies are most likely life-threatening, and you know to avoid these foods. The things you miss from these foods are the heart-healthy fats. Fortunately, there are other sources for these oils. To replace nuts and peanuts, use avocados or olives. (Yes, olives are high-salt, but you can have them occasionally.) And, of course, extra virgin olive oil is chock-full of monounsaturated, heart-healthy fat. It is a little more challenging to get the exact type of omega-3 fats you need from vegetable sources instead of fish. But you can get other omega-3s in walnuts. Omega-3s are also present in flax, but I am not a fan of flax, because of the high oxidative potential of its fats. You will also find small amounts of omega-3s in cruciferous vegetables (including broccoli, cauliflower, and Brussels sprouts), chia seeds, and hummus (if the sesame seeds are used as part of the starting raw materials—and I do understand that some people with nut allergies are also allergic to sesame seeds).

Dairy can be challenging. None of the replacement foods has exactly the right combination of ingredients to give the full benefit. And there has never been a research study to show whether dairy substitutes work as well in DASH as real dairy foods do. If you have a true allergy, of course you need to avoid dairy. You can substitute soy milk or almond milk for regular milk. There are cheeses and yogurts that are also dairy-free. Yes, these are processed foods, but they can be helpful in providing substitutes for milk that are rich in calcium and vitamin D. However, almond milk is very low in protein, and real milk proteins are especially powerful for preserving and building muscle. If you are having almond milk, perhaps consider adding some eggs or egg whites to the same meal, to replace the milk protein with another high-quality protein. And focus on getting lots of green leafy vegetables and cruciferous vegetables, which are good sources of calcium. Many people are only sensitive to the lactose in dairy products. You can add enzyme drops to milk to predigest the lactose or buy milk that already has the enzyme added. And yogurt and most cheeses have very little or no lactose. When yogurt is made, lactose is converted into lactic acid during the fermentation process. And the good bacteria in the yogurt may

(continued)

help boost your ability to digest lactose in other foods. During the process of making cheese, most of the lactose goes out with the whey (remember Miss Muffet's curds and whey?). And milk is much easier to digest after being heated (such as in hot chocolate or lattes), so this is another way to see if you can expand the types of dairy foods you can tolerate. But, by all means, feel free to substitute non-dairy alternatives, if you have allergies or intolerances to dairy.

Just as with wheat, it is very easy to eliminate corn, including any hidden sources, by following the DASH Diet Younger You program. Whole foods, unprocessed or only minimally processed, will help you avoid this potential allergen. My symptoms are puffiness and a runny nose, so this is a mild allergy for me. Many people have more severe allergies and need to completely avoid corn, which, again, is quite easy. You can substitute non-corn-based tortillas in any of the recipes.

If you have an allergy to penicillin, you will probably also be sensitive to mold. If you think you aren't eating moldy foods, think again. Blue cheese and goat cheese are everywhere. Mushrooms are in so many elegant dishes. And you will notice that I have included few of these very common foods in any of my recipes. That doesn't mean that you can't choose them, but I have accommodated this very common but relatively unknown allergy, which can cause puffiness and blurry thinking. Mold is so pervasive, in the air and in our food, that the allergy is underrecognized. You just know that occasionally, or frequently, you seem to have a very puffy face and clogged sinuses.

14 Days of Menu Ideas for Vegetarian Meals

(Recipes found in the book are marked with *.)

Week 1, Monday

Breakfast

Hard-boiled egg
1 slice light whole wheat toast with 1 teaspoon jam
4 fluid ounces orange juice
Latte (made with 8 fluid ounces nonfat milk)

Lunch

PB&J: 2 tablespoons natural peanut butter and 1 tablespoon
    jam on 2 slices light whole wheat bread
1 medium sliced tomato, or 8 grape tomatoes
½ cup Traditional Coleslaw*
1 small Granny Smith apple
Glass of water with lemon slices

Snack

8 fluid ounces Nonfat Fruit-Flavored Yogurt*
1 ounce almonds

Dinner

Garbanzo Bean Curry with Potatoes*
Salad
Glass of red wine

Week 1, Tuesday

Breakfast

1 ounce whole wheat cereal
8 fluid ounces nonfat milk
4 ounces raspberries
4 fluid ounces orange juice

Lunch

Santa Fe Lentils in Tortillas,* in whole wheat or corn
    tortillas, or on the salad
Side salad, with Ranch Dressing*
8 fluid ounces nonfat milk
4 ounces fresh pineapple slices
Glass of water with lemon slices

Snack

Plum
1 ounce reduced-fat cheese

Dinner

Faux Pasta e Fagioli alla Venezia*
Stone Fruit Salad*
Glass of red wine

Week 1, Wednesday

Breakfast

1 ounce cashews
4 ounces strawberries
4 fluid ounces low-sodium tomato juice
Hot chocolate (made with 8 fluid ounces nonfat milk)

Lunch

New Vegetable Bean Salad*
Carrot sticks
1 ounce reduced-fat cheese
Nectarine
Glass of water with orange slices

Snack

Small pear
8 fluid ounces Nonfat Fruit-Flavored Yogurt*

Dinner

Rice with Black-Eyed Peas, Lentils, and Tomatoes*
Mango Walnut Salad* with Citrus Vinaigrette*
Glass of red wine

Week 1, Thursday

Breakfast

Fabulous Oatmeal*
8 fluid ounces nonfat milk
½ medium banana
4 fluid ounces orange juice

Lunch

Hummus* sandwich on 1 whole wheat pita, topped with
    cucumbers, bell pepper slices, and tomato slices
Small peach
Glass of water with orange slices

Snack

Small apple, sliced and dipped in 2 tablespoons peanut butter

Dinner

Zucchini and Tomato Frittata*
Salad: frisée lettuce, topped with Citrus Vinaigrette* and
    1 ounce pine nuts
Glass of red wine

Week 1, Friday

Breakfast

PB&J: 2 tablespoons natural peanut butter and 1 tablespoon
    jam on 2 slices light whole wheat toast
4 fluid ounces apple juice
Latte (made with 8 fluid ounces nonfat milk)
Plum

Lunch

Yellow Split Pea Soup with Sweet Potatoes and Mustard
    Greens*
Side salad with Citrus Vinaigrette*
Apple
Glass of water with lemon slices

Snack

1½ cups red grapes
1 ounce reduced-fat cheese

Dinner

Pesto Pizza*
Salad topped with garbanzo beans and Ranch
    Dressing*
Glass of red wine

Week 1, Saturday

Breakfast

Curried Eggs*
Sliced tomatoes
1 slice light whole wheat toast with 1 teaspoon jam
8 fluid ounces Nonfat Fruit-Flavored Yogurt*
4 fluid ounces pineapple juice

Lunch

Texas Caviar* on salad, sprinkled with 1 ounce reduced-fat
   cheese
4 ounces mango slices
Glass of water with cucumber slices

Snack

1 ounce Spicy Roasted Nuts* (see variation in Spiced Roasted
   Chickpeas recipe)
Fuji apple

Dinner

Tomato Pasta Primavera*
Hearty Dinner Salad* with Italian Dressing*
Glass of red wine

Week 1, Sunday

Breakfast

Omelet with Bell Peppers, Onions, and Tomatoes*
1 slice raisin bread toast
4 fluid ounces orange juice
4 ounces blueberries
Latte (made with 8 fluid ounces nonfat milk)

Lunch

BBQ'd Lentils* topped with 1 ounce reduced-fat cheese
Ear of sweet corn
4 ounces strawberries
Glass of water with lemon slices

Snack

Roasted Cauliflower "Popcorn"*

Dinner

Risotto with Lentils, Mushrooms, Leeks, and Pine Nuts*
Hearty Dinner Salad* with Italian Dressing*

Week 2, Monday

Breakfast

½ cup cooked oatmeal, mixed with ½ cup Unsweetened
    Applesauce*
8 fluid ounces nonfat milk
½ medium banana
4 fluid ounces orange juice

Lunch

Caprese Grilled Cheese Sandwich* (or Caprese Salad* on top
    of the field greens, if you don't want the bread)
Field greens salad with Citrus Vinaigrette*
½ cup sliced raw zucchini or cucumbers
Glass of water with lemon slices
Small peach

Snack

1 ounce almonds
4 ounces strawberries

Dinner

Creamy Rice with Fresh Peas*
Braised Radishes*
Stone Fruit Salad*
Glass of red wine

Week 2, Tuesday

Breakfast

1 ounce Homemade Granola*
8 fluid ounces nonfat milk
¼ cup raisins
4 fluid ounces pineapple juice
4 ounces cantaloupe

Lunch

New Vegetable Bean Salad*
2 kiwifruits
8 fluid ounces Nonfat Fruit-Flavored Yogurt*
Glass of water with orange slices

Snack

Salt-Free Pickles*
Hard-boiled egg

Dinner

Pasta and Broccoli*
Caprese Salad*
Glass of red wine

Week 2, Wednesday

Breakfast

Mini Egg Scramble* or Tofu Scramble*
1 slice light whole wheat toast with 1 teaspoon jam
4 fluid ounces low-sodium tomato juice
4 ounces strawberries
Latte (made with 8 fluid ounces nonfat milk)

Lunch

Lentil Confetti Salad*
Plum
Glass of water with lemon slices

Snack

Apple
1 ounce reduced-fat cheese

Dinner

Kung Pao Chicken* (or Kung Pao Tofu* variation)
Asian Coleslaw*
Glass of red wine

Week 2, Thursday

Breakfast

Hard-boiled egg

1 ounce cashews

4 ounces raspberries

Hot chocolate (made with 8 fluid ounces nonfat milk)

Lunch

Caesar's Egg Salad Sandwich* (alternately, tomato stuffed
    with Caesar's Egg Salad)

Carrot sticks

Cucumber slices

Plum

Snack

Baked Kale Chips*

Dinner

Southern Corn Casserole*

Hearty Dinner Salad*

Glass of red wine

Week 2, Friday

Breakfast

Southwestern Omelet*

4 fluid ounces orange juice

Latte (made with 8 fluid ounces nonfat milk)

Lunch

Salade Niçoise with Garbanzo Beans*
1½ cups red grapes
Glass of water with lemon slices

Snack

8 fluid ounces Nonfat Fruit-Flavored Yogurt*
1 ounce cashews

Dinner

South of the Border Tofu Enchiladas*
Salad with Citrus Vinaigrette*
Glass of white wine

Week 2, Saturday

Breakfast

½ cup cooked oatmeal
4 ounces blueberries
Hard-boiled egg
4 fluid ounces orange juice
Latte (made with 8 fluid ounces nonfat milk)

Lunch

PB&J: 2 tablespoons natural peanut butter and 1 tablespoon
    jam on 2 slices light whole wheat bread
8 grape tomatoes
Carrot sticks
Glass of water with orange slices
Apple

Snack

Avocado Deviled Eggs*
1 ounce almonds

Dinner

Whole wheat pasta and Pesto*
Caprese Salad* with Italian Dressing*
Glass of red wine

Week 2, Sunday

Breakfast

Zucchini and Tomato Frittata*
4 fluid ounces cranberry juice
8 fluid ounces nonfat milk

Lunch

Zucchini Lasagna*
Side salad with Italian Dressing*
Sliced pear
Glass of water with orange slices

Snack

Spicy Roasted Edamame*
8 fluid ounces Nonfat Fruit-Flavored Yogurt*

Dinner

Vegetarian Chili*
Glass of red wine

7 Days of Menu Ideas for Fish and Poultry Lovers

Monday

Breakfast

1 Shredded Wheat biscuit
8 fluid ounces nonfat milk
4 ounces strawberries
4 fluid ounces orange juice

Lunch

Tuna salad fish sandwich or tuna-stuffed tomato
Carrot sticks
Celery sticks
Radishes
Plum
Glass of water with orange slices

Snack

Small apple, sliced and dipped in 2 tablespoons peanut butter

Dinner

Simple Baked Salmon*
Roasted Brussels Sprouts with Balsamic Vinegar and Pine Nuts*
Radicchio salad with Citrus Vinaigrette*
Glass of white wine

Tuesday

Breakfast

Scrambled eggs (or Mini Egg Scramble* or Tofu Scramble*
    variation)
4 fluid ounces orange juice

Latte (made with 8 fluid ounces nonfat milk)
Cantaloupe wedge

Lunch

Lunch Base Salad* topped with Simple Baked Salmon* (left
    over from dinner on Monday night) and Citrus Vinaigrette*
Nectarine
Glass of water with orange slices

Snack

8 grape tomatoes
1 ounce cashews

Dinner

Kung Pao Chicken* (or Kung Pao Tofu* variation)
Romaine topped with tangerine slices and sliced almonds,
    with Citrus Vinaigrette*
Glass of red wine

Wednesday

Breakfast

½ cup cooked oatmeal
½ banana, mashed and mixed into the oatmeal
8 fluid ounces nonfat milk
4 fluid ounces cran-raspberry juice

Lunch

Berry Good Salad with Grilled Chicken* (or Berry Good
    Salad with Tofu* variation)
Plum
Glass of water with lemon slices

Snack

Peach

Hard-boiled egg

Dinner

Skillet BBQ'd Chicken*

Ear of sweet corn

Sliced green beans

Glass of red wine

Thursday

Breakfast

1 or 2 hard-boiled eggs

4 ounces strawberries

4 fluid ounces orange juice

Hot chocolate (made with 8 fluid ounces nonfat milk)

Lunch

Turkey and reduced-fat Swiss cheese sandwich on light whole
    wheat bread, topped with lettuce slices and sliced tomato
    (2–4 ounces turkey, 1 slice Swiss cheese)

Salt-Free Pickles*

Carrot slices

Apple

Snack

Baked Kale Chips*

Dinner

Baked Tilapia* with Peach Salsa*

Steamed broccoli
Side salad with Citrus Vinaigrette*
Glass of white wine

Friday

Breakfast

1 ounce whole grain cereal
8 fluid ounces nonfat milk
4 ounces raspberries
4 fluid ounces orange juice

Lunch

Curried Chicken Salad*
Tangerine
Glass of water with lemon slices

Snack

Peach
1 ounce almonds

Dinner

Super-Quick Chicken Stir-Fry*
Glass of red wine

Saturday

Breakfast

PB&J: 2 tablespoons natural peanut butter and 1 tablespoon
    jam on 2 slices light whole wheat bread
4 fluid ounces orange juice
Latte (made with 8 fluid ounces nonfat milk)

Lunch

Salade Niçoise*
Peach
Glass of water with lemon slices

Snack

Avocado Deviled Eggs*

Dinner

Lemon Chicken Breasts*
Roasted Brussels Sprouts with Balsamic Vinegar
    and Pine Nuts*
Glass of red wine

Sunday

Breakfast

Omelet with Bell Peppers, Onions, and Tomatoes*
Cantaloupe wedge
4 fluid ounces low-sodium tomato juice
Latte (made with 8 fluid ounces nonfat milk)

Lunch

Grilled Napa Chicken Sandwich*
Sliced cucumbers
1½ cups red grapes
Glass of water with lemon slices

Snack

Small apple, sliced and dipped in 2 tablespoons natural peanut
    butter

Dinner

Caribbean Chicken*
Steamed asparagus
Hearty Dinner Salad* with Citrus Vinaigrette*
Glass of red wine

7 Days of Menu Ideas for Meat Lovers (Includes Chicken and Fish)

Monday

Breakfast

Scrambled eggs (or Mini Egg Scramble* or Tofu Scramble*
    variation)
1 slice light whole wheat toast with 1 teaspoon jam
4 fluid ounces orange juice
Hot chocolate (made with 8 fluid ounces nonfat milk)

Lunch

Ham and reduced-fat Swiss cheese roll-up or sandwich on
    light whole wheat bread, topped with lettuce, sliced
    tomato, and mustard
Carrot slices
1 cup Asian Coleslaw*
Orange
Glass of water with lemon slices

Snack

Peach
10 peanuts in shell (20 individual peanuts)

Dinner

Halibut with Salted Black Beans and Chilies*
1 cup steamed broccoli
Greek Pepper Salad*
Glass of red wine

Tuesday

Breakfast

1 ounce bran cereal
8 fluid ounces milk
4 ounces raspberries
4 fluid ounces orange-banana juice

Lunch

Lunch Base Salad* topped with grilled chicken
Plum
Glass of water with cucumber slices

Snack

8 fluid ounces Nonfat Fruit-Flavored Yogurt*
1 ounce almonds

Dinner

Peach and Balsamic Glazed Pork Chops*
Farmer's Salad*
Glass of red wine

Wednesday

Breakfast

1 or 2 hard-boiled eggs
4 ounces strawberries
1 ounce cashews
4 ounces orange juice
Latte (made with 8 fluid ounces nonfat milk)

Lunch

Lean roast beef and reduced-fat provolone cheese roll-up
    or sandwich on light whole wheat bread, topped
    with lettuce, sliced tomato, and mustard
Waldorf Salad*
Plum
Glass of water with cucumber slices

Snack

¼ cup Guacamole*
Raw veggies, such as sliced bell peppers, carrots, cucumbers,
    and celery

Dinner

Lemon Chicken Breasts*
Risotto with Lentils, Mushrooms, Leeks, and Pine Nuts*
Glass of red wine

Thursday

Breakfast

½ cup cooked oatmeal, mixed with ½ cup
Unsweetened Applesauce,* sprinkled
with cinnamon
8 fluid ounces nonfat milk
½ banana
4 fluid ounces orange juice

Lunch

Grilled Cheese Sandwich with Pesto and Tomato*
Side salad with Italian Dressing*
Nectarine
Glass of water with lemon slices

Snack

8 fluid ounces Nonfat Fruit-Flavored Yogurt*
Pear

Dinner

Steak and Roasted Vegetable Salad*
Glass of red wine

Friday

Breakfast

Mini Egg Scramble* (or Tofu Scramble* variation)
4 ounces strawberries
Cantaloupe wedge
Hot chocolate (made with 8 fluid ounces nonfat
milk)

Lunch

PB&J: 2 tablespoons natural peanut butter and 1 tablespoon
 jam on 2 slices light whole wheat bread
Asian Coleslaw*
1½ cups red grapes
Glass of water with lemon slices

Snack

Orange
1 ounce walnuts

Dinner

Kung Pao Chicken* (or Kung Pao Tofu* variation)
Glass of red wine

Saturday

Breakfast

Curried Eggs*
1 slice whole wheat toast with 1 teaspoon jam
4 ounces pineapple slices
4 fluid ounces orange juice
Latte (made with 8 fluid ounces nonfat milk)

Lunch

Texas Caviar* on Lunch Base Salad*
Apple
Glass of water with cucumber slices

Snack

¼ cup Hummus*
Sliced bell peppers

Dinner

Caribbean Chicken*
Southern Corn Casserole*
Side salad with Citrus Vinaigrette*
Glass of red wine

Sunday

Breakfast

1 ounce whole wheat cereal
8 fluid ounces nonfat milk
4 ounces raspberries
4 fluid ounces orange juice

Lunch

Grilled Chicken Caprese Sandwich*
Asian Coleslaw*
Peach
Glass of water with orange slices

Snack

Apple
1 ounce cashews

Dinner

Carnitas*
Hearty Dinner Salad* with Citrus Vinaigrette*
Texas Caviar*
Glass of red wine

Change Your Relationship with Food to Change Your Body

We have bought into the idea that to eat healthfully, we need to analyze food labels, count calories and fat grams, cut back on protein, and pump up the grains. Not to mention tracking our activity calories every moment of the day. It can be hard to break away from those old patterns. However, they haven't gotten you where you want to be.

A newer, fresher way to think about food is to enjoy it! What a concept. You are going to love eating more fresh fruits and vegetables. You will pair them up with protein-rich foods, including nuts, some fresh fish, lots of beans. You'll also enjoy dairy foods—so satisfying. Add in some whole grains and heart-healthy fats and you are eating wonderfully clean. You will stop eating when you are naturally satisfied. How lovely!

You don't have to count calories when you follow the DASH Diet Younger You program. Fill at least half of your plate with veggies and add a side salad with *real* dressing (not fat-free). Have something protein-rich, such as one of my fabulous bean dishes or some fresh wild salmon with lemon. Include a small portion of grains (or not—it's up to you). For dessert, try some yogurt and fresh fruit. The proteins and heart-healthy fats keep you satisfied longer so you aren't craving more food an hour later. The fruits and vegetables are bulky and filling so you naturally avoid overeating. If you absolutely have to track something, track your servings from each of the food groups while you become accustomed to your new food pattern, using our chart in Appendix D.

(continued)

The same is true for activity. Don't track your calories burned; that tends to make people think they can eat more. Do activity because it makes you feel good. Walking brightens your mood. Dancing is fun. Strength training makes your body feel (and actually become) younger.

So give up your apps, your online tracking, your magnifying glass for reading labels, and enjoy fresh, delightful, clean eating and being more active. It will make you younger!

CHAPTER 8

Younger You Recipes

To help you enjoy eating the DASH Diet Younger You way, I have included many of my favorite recipes. Some of these were developed when I taught Introductory Food Science at the University of Illinois at Chicago. They were hands-on tested, and often made more interesting, by many students, with varying levels of culinary skills and with a variety of ethnic and cultural food habits. I hope you will find lots of new ideas here.

Think of the recipes as suggestions instead of rigid requirements. Then you will be able to create your own special meals that are perfect for your personal tastes.

Enjoy healthy eating!

Breakfast

Zucchini and Tomato Frittata

6 large eggs
2 leaves basil, thinly sliced
1 teaspoon fresh oregano, minced
1 tablespoon extra virgin olive oil
1 small zucchini, sliced
1 small onion, thinly sliced
1 cup grape tomatoes, halved, or 1 medium flavorful tomato, diced
1 small clove garlic, minced
2 tablespoons Parmesan

Preheat the broiler.

In a medium bowl, lightly whisk the eggs. Add the basil and oregano and stir.

Heat the oil in an oven-safe medium sauté pan over medium heat. Add the zucchini and onion and sauté for 5 minutes, stirring occasionally. Stir in the tomatoes and garlic and sauté for 1–2 minutes, until softened. Pour the egg mixture into the sauté pan and stir. Allow the edges of the frittata to set. Use a spatula to lift the edges and separate slightly in the interior, allowing the eggs to thicken throughout. Sprinkle with the cheese. Brown under the broiler for 2–3 minutes. Serve immediately.

Makes 6 servings.

Southwestern Omelet

1 tablespoon extra virgin olive oil or butter
½ cup sliced red bell (sweet) pepper (freeze the rest of the pepper for another day or refrigerate for use in a salad)
½ cup grape tomatoes, halved, or 1 small flavorful tomato, diced
1 small onion, diced

1 small jalapeño pepper, seeds and ribs removed, minced
4 large eggs
¼ cup reduced-fat Monterey Jack cheese

Heat the oil or butter in a small skillet over medium heat. Add the pepper, tomato, onion, and jalapeño and sauté about 2 minutes until softened. In a small bowl, whisk the eggs. Add the eggs to the skillet and cook until the edges are set, about 15 seconds. With a spatula, lift the edges of the egg so the uncooked liquid can flow underneath. Continue cooking, lifting the edges about every 15 seconds, until the omelet is set, about 1½ minutes total.

Remove from the heat. Sprinkle the cheese over the top of the omelet. Tilt the pan slightly and use the spatula to help the omelet fold over on itself. Slide onto a plate and serve.

Makes 2 servings.

Hate the Heat? Variation

Omelet with Bell Peppers, Onions, and Tomatoes

For a mild take on the spicy Southwestern Omelet, substitute ½ cup green or orange bell pepper for the jalapeño and eliminate the cheese.

Mini Egg Scramble

Need a quick and healthy breakfast? Try this mini scramble the next time you're in a rush!

1 large egg
½ teaspoon butter

In a small glass bowl, whisk the egg until it is airy. Add the butter. Microwave on high for 2 minutes. Serve immediately. If you prefer, use a small sauté pan, melt the butter first, then add the egg, and use a spatula to separate and allow to cook through, about every 15 seconds. When the egg is thoroughly cooked, remove it from the heat and serve.

You could also double this recipe for a larger breakfast, and add a little milk to make it creamier, especially if you are cooking it in a sauté pan.

Makes 1 serving.

Don't Fear the Microwave

Yes, it is perfectly safe. Contrary to opinions you may have read on the Internet, the microwave oven does not change the molecular structure of water. It changes the structure of the food by cooking, in the same way that heating by any means changes food.

Fabulous Oatmeal

3½ cups hot tap water
1 cup steel-cut (Irish) oats
¼ cup half-and-half
3 tablespoons (packed) brown sugar
½ teaspoon ground cinnamon
⅛ teaspoon ground ginger
⅛ teaspoon ground allspice
1 teaspoon vanilla extract
¼ cup currants or raisins

In a heavy-bottomed saucepan, bring the water to a boil.

Add the oats, reduce the heat, and simmer, stirring occasionally, until the oatmeal is thick and tender, about 35 minutes. During the last

10 minutes of cooking, stir frequently to prevent the oatmeal from scorching.

Stir in the remaining ingredients, taste, and adjust the flavors per your own taste preference. Serve immediately.

Makes 8 servings.

Curried Eggs

2 tablespoons extra virgin olive oil
1 medium onion, diced
½ small jalapeño pepper, seeds and ribs removed, minced
2 cloves garlic, minced
2 teaspoons fresh gingerroot, minced
¼ teaspoon ground coriander
¼ teaspoon ground cayenne pepper
1 tablespoon cilantro, minced
8 eggs

Heat the oil in a medium skillet over medium heat. Add the onion and jalapeño and sauté about 5 minutes, stirring occasionally with a spatula. Add the garlic, ginger, coriander, cayenne pepper, and cilantro and sauté about 1 minute. Add the eggs and stir frequently to form soft curds, until the eggs are firmly set. Serve immediately.

Makes 4 servings.

Tofu Scramble

This is a vegan version of scrambled eggs, a recipe developed by one of my student dietitians at the University of Illinois at Chicago, Stephanie Brendle. It is very high-flavor and has a good yellow color, thanks to the turmeric and the sweet corn. Everyone in our class loved this dish!

2 tablespoons extra virgin olive oil
2–3 scallions (green onions), chopped
½ medium jalapeño pepper, seeds and ribs removed, minced
3 cloves garlic
½ teaspoon ground ginger
1 teaspoon ground coriander
¼ teaspoon ground cayenne pepper
1 tablespoon fresh cilantro, minced
1 pound extra-firm tofu, drained
7–9 mushrooms, chopped
½ cup yellow bell pepper, seeds and ribs removed, chopped
¼ teaspoon salt
Dash freshly ground black pepper
⅛ teaspoon turmeric
½ cup frozen corn
1 tomato, chopped
½ teaspoon curry powder
1 tablespoon low-sodium soy sauce
¼ cup chopped fresh Italian parsley

Heat the oil in a medium skillet over medium heat. Add the scallions and jalapeño and sauté about 5 minutes. Add the garlic, ginger, coriander, cayenne pepper, and cilantro and sauté about 1 minute. Crumble the tofu into the pan, stirring to break it up, add the rest of the ingredients except the parsley, and mix well to mingle the flavors, until heated through. Turn out onto a serving plate and top with the parsley. Serve immediately.

Makes 4 servings.

Homemade Granola

2 tablespoons maple syrup
2 tablespoons water
1 tablespoon canola oil
1 teaspoon ground cinnamon
4 cups old-fashioned (rolled) oats

1 cup golden raisins
¼ cup chopped almonds

Preheat the oven to 300°F.

In a large bowl, whisk together the maple syrup, water, oil, and cinnamon. Add the oats and mix until lightly coated. Spread evenly on a large rimmed baking sheet.

Bake, stirring occasionally and bringing the toasted edges in toward the center, until the oats are evenly crisp, about 40 minutes. Remove from the oven and stir in the raisins and almonds. Let cool completely. Store in an airtight container up to 2 weeks.

For each serving, scoop ½ cup of granola into a bowl and add milk.

Makes 10 servings.

Lunch

Caesar's Egg Salad Sandwich

⅓ cup mayonnaise
2½ tablespoons grated Parmesan
2 teaspoons minced garlic
1 teaspoon lemon juice
1 teaspoon Worcestershire sauce (optional)
¼ teaspoon hot pepper sauce, such as Tabasco
¼ teaspoon freshly ground white pepper
Dash salt
4 teaspoons extra virgin olive oil
8 hard-boiled eggs, diced
4 whole wheat pita bread rounds
2 cups romaine, shredded
4 teaspoons chopped Italian parsley (optional)

Blend the mayonnaise, Parmesan, garlic, lemon juice, Worcestershire sauce (if using), hot pepper sauce, pepper, and salt. When combined, drizzle in the olive oil, whisking constantly.

Fold in the diced eggs. Cover and refrigerate until ready to serve.

To serve, fill each pita round with about ½ cup romaine and ½ cup egg salad.

Sprinkle each with 1 teaspoon parsley, if desired.

Makes 4 servings.

Lunch Base Salad

These ingredients are ideas for a high-impact salad that is delicious and packed with antioxidants, vitamins, and minerals. Don't get stuck on just lettuce, especially if you are making a lunchtime main dish salad—you need it to energize you all afternoon. Pack it full of wonderful high-flavor and high-color foods. You get to decide the ratios. You might cut up some of the ingredients over the weekend and refrigerate them in airtight containers to make it easier to have variety in your salads during the week.

Lettuce (romaine and/or iceberg)
Grated carrots
Bell pepper strips
Sunflower seeds and/or pine nuts
Cucumber slices
Grape tomatoes
Hard-boiled egg slices
Sliced mushrooms
Sliced red cabbage
Celery slices

Grilled Cheese Sandwich with Pesto and Tomato

How can you make the old standby into a standout? Pesto is the secret ingredient for high flavor.

2 tablespoons Pesto (page 183)
2 slices light whole wheat bread

2 slices reduced-fat Swiss cheese
1 flavorful tomato, sliced

Spread 1 tablespoon of the pesto on each slice of bread and top each with a slice of Swiss cheese. Place the sliced tomato on top of the cheese on one of the pieces of bread. Place both pieces of bread on the rack in a toaster oven and toast until the cheese starts to melt. Turn the slice of toast without the tomatoes facedown on the other slice. Serve immediately.

Makes 1 serving.

Caprese Grilled Cheese Sandwich

For a Caprese version of the Grilled Cheese Sandwich with Pesto and Tomato, omit the pesto; substitute buffalo mozzarella for the Swiss cheese, cutting the mozzarella into ¼-inch-thick slices for both slices of bread; top one with the sliced tomato. After toasting, top the slice with the tomato with thinly sliced basil and drizzle with extra virgin olive oil and balsamic vinegar. Top with the second piece of toast.

Lentil Confetti Salad

4 cups water
1 cup lentils, rinsed
1 cup long-grain brown rice
1 large tomato, diced
½ cup red onion, finely diced
½ cup celery, chopped
¼ cup pimento-stuffed olives, sliced
¼ cup green bell pepper, diced medium
1 tablespoon fresh Italian parsley, chopped
½ cup Italian Dressing (page 182)

In a saucepan, pour the water over the lentils and rice, bring to a boil, cover, and simmer 20 minutes, or until the lentils are tender.

Combine the drained lentils and rice with all the vegetables. Sprinkle with the parsley and toss lightly with the dressing.

Makes 2 servings.

Recipe adapted from the USA Dry Pea & Lentil Council.

Santa Fe Lentils in Tortillas

Lentil Filling:

1 cup lentils, rinsed
1 medium red bell pepper, diced
1 medium green bell pepper, diced
1 medium jalapeño pepper, seeds and ribs removed, finely diced
1 can (14½ fluid ounces) vegetable broth (or Homemade Vegetable Broth, page 133)
¼ cup finely diced onion
2 cloves garlic, minced
1 teaspoon ground cumin
1 teaspoon fresh oregano leaves, minced
1 teaspoon salt
1 cup frozen corn

Tortillas and Toppings:

16 corn tortillas
8 ounces reduced-fat shredded Colby-Jack cheese
2 cups chopped lettuce
2 medium flavorful tomatoes, diced, or 2 cups quartered cherry tomatoes

In a medium saucepan, combine the lentils with the remaining filling ingredients. Heat to boiling. Reduce the heat, cover, and simmer until the lentils are very soft, 25–30 minutes.

Place ½ cup of the lentil mixture on each tortilla; garnish with cheese, lettuce, and tomatoes to taste; and roll. The lentils may also be served on lettuce, as a salad, for a lighter version.

Makes 8 servings (2 tortillas per person).

Recipe adapted from the USA Dry Pea & Lentil Council.

Homemade Vegetable Broth

Want to make your own vegetable broth? This is a high-flavor version that you can use as a substitute in any recipe calling for chicken or beef stock or broth.

1 tablespoon vegetable oil (preferably extra virgin olive oil)
1 medium yellow onion, chopped
1 medium leek, rinsed well and chopped
1 clove garlic, minced
2 medium carrots, chopped
1 medium celery rib, chopped
4½ quarts water
4 sprigs fresh Italian parsley
½ teaspoon black peppercorns
¼ teaspoon dried thyme
1 bay leaf

Heat the oil in a large stockpot over medium heat. Add the onion, leek, garlic, carrots, and celery and cook, stirring occasionally, until softened, about 5 minutes.

Add the water, increase the heat under the pot, and bring just to a boil. Reduce the heat to low. Add the parsley, peppercorns, thyme, and bay leaf. Simmer, uncovered, about 45 minutes.

Using a hand blender (or a regular blender in batches), blend until smooth.

The broth can be refrigerated for up to 3 days or transferred to airtight containers and frozen for up to 3 months.

Makes about 16 cups.

Berry Good Salad with Grilled Chicken

1 tablespoon paprika
2 teaspoons dried thyme
2 teaspoons dried oregano
1 teaspoon feshly ground black pepper
1 teaspoon garlic powder
1 teaspoon onion powder
¼ teaspoon ground cayenne pepper
4 boneless, skinless chicken breasts (4 ounces each)
1 tablespoon extra virgin olive oil
2–3 cups lettuce mix (your preferences)
2 medium flavorful tomatoes, cut into wedges, or substitute
    20 grape tomatoes
½ cup shredded red cabbage
½ cup shredded carrots
1 cup sliced strawberries
1 cup red raspberries
1 cup blueberries
Dijon Vinaigrette (page 182)

Combine the paprika, thyme, oregano, pepper, garlic powder, onion powder, and cayenne pepper in a small bowl. Place in a thin layer on a small plate. Rinse the chicken breasts and blot dry with a paper towel. Coat each side of the chicken breasts with the spice mixture. Heat the oil in a skillet over medium-high heat. Sear both sides of the chicken, reduce heat to medium, and cook 2–3 minutes per side, until cooked through. (Alternately, the chicken can be cooked on a grill, searing first, then cooking over medium heat, about 2–3 minutes per side, until cooked through.) Let cool a few minutes, then slice crosswise into 1-inch strips.

Arrange your lettuce on plates and cover with tomatoes, red cabbage, and shredded carrots. Place the chicken strips on each salad and top with a variety of the berries. Dress with the vinaigrette.

Makes 4 servings.

Berry Good Salad with Tofu

Make this delicious salad vegetarian by substituting 1 pound of silken tofu for the chicken. Add 1 medium thinly sliced onion to the skillet before adding the tofu. Sauté the onion for 5 minutes, then add the spice mixture and blend well. Break up the tofu and add to the pan, stirring to break up further and to mingle the flavors. When fully heated, complete as for chicken.

BBQ'd Lentils

Yes, this recipe calls for more processed ingredients than I would typically use, but it's an easy and delicious way to get more protein-rich and fiberful lentils into your diet. If you hate the idea of using store-bought ketchup, you can substitute fresh flavorful tomatoes and additional tomato sauce. And this is a fun recipe, making a large number of servings so you can have meals for several days without cooking again, or freeze for later use.

2½ cups lentils, rinsed
5 cups water
½ cup molasses
2 tablespoons (packed) brown sugar
1 tablespoon apple cider vinegar
½ cup ketchup
1 teaspoon dry mustard
1 teaspoon Worcestershire sauce
1 can (16 fluid ounces) tomato sauce
1 small onion, diced

Preheat the oven to 350°F.

In a saucepan, add the lentils to the water, bring to a boil, and simmer for 30 minutes, or until tender but still whole.

Add the remaining ingredients to the cooked lentils, pour into a 9-by-13-inch baking dish, and bake for 45 minutes.

Makes 16 servings.

Recipe adapted from the USA Dry Pea & Lentil Council.

Grilled Chicken Caprese Sandwich

4 skinless, boneless chicken breast halves (4 ounces each), either thin-cut or pounded to a uniform thickness (make extra, if desired, to freeze for salads)
4 whole wheat hamburger buns (optional)
2 medium flavorful tomatoes, sliced
1 ball (8 ounces) buffalo mozzarella, cut into ¼-inch-thick slices
4 leaves basil, thinly sliced
Extra virgin olive oil
Balsamic vinegar

Heat a grill to high. Sear the chicken on each side, turn the heat down to medium, and cook the chicken thoroughly, about 2–3 minutes per side.

Place each cooked chicken breast half on top of the bottom part of a bun, if using. Top with 1 tomato slice, 1 slice mozzarella, 1 additional tomato slice, and some of the basil. Drizzle with olive oil and balsamic vinegar. Top with the other half of the bun. Alternatively, you could skip the bun and cut the chicken into bite-sized pieces to serve over a green salad. If you don't have a grill, you can pan-broil the chicken in a medium sauté pan with 1 tablespoon olive oil.

Makes 4 servings.

Grilled Napa Chicken Sandwich

For a Napa-inspired variation, top the chicken with 2 slices avocado, 2 tablespoons black olives, and Pesto (page 183) instead of the tomatoes and mozzarella.

Curried Chicken Salad

½ cup mayonnaise or plain low-fat Greek yogurt
½ teaspoon curry powder
½ teaspoon cayenne pepper
¼ teaspoon freshly ground black pepper
2 skinless, boneless chicken breasts (4 ounces each), poached, and cut into 1-inch pieces
1 stalk celery, chopped
1 medium red apple, diced (don't peel)
½ cup chopped walnuts
½ cup raisins

Mix the mayonnaise or yogurt and the spices. Add the remaining ingredients and mix well to coat with the mayonnaise mixture. Refrigerate at least 30 minutes. Serve chilled.

Makes 2–3 servings.

Snacks

Avocado Deviled Eggs

Green eggs and…I've taken the traditional deviled egg recipe and given it a healthy makeover by using avocado—which is rich in good fats and fiber—instead of mayonnaise. If you love this recipe, double it, because it keeps well in the fridge and it makes an easy and healthy snack to have on hand.

6 hard-boiled eggs
½ cup mashed avocado
1 teaspoon white vinegar
1 teaspoon Tabasco sauce
1 teaspoon yellow or Dijon mustard
Dash freshly ground black pepper
Paprika

Slice eggs in half lengthwise and remove yolks to a small bowl. In the small bowl, combine the yolks, avocado, vinegar, Tabasco, mustard, and pepper and mash with a pastry cutter or fork until well blended. Spoon the mixture into the egg white halves, or use a pastry bag to fill. Sprinkle with paprika. Serve chilled.

Makes 6 servings (2 egg halves per serving).

Spiced Roasted Chickpeas

3 cups canned garbanzo beans (chickpeas), or cooked from dry
   (page 139)
2 tablespoons extra virgin olive oil
1 teaspoon ground cumin
1 teaspoon chili powder
½ teaspoon cayenne pepper

Preheat the oven to 400°F. Mix all the ingredients gently in a mixing bowl, coating the beans well with the seasonings. Put the beans into a rectangular glass casserole or onto a cookie sheet lined with nonstick aluminum foil. (The nonstick aluminum foil makes for easy cleanup. No, I don't believe there is any connection between aluminum and Alzheimer's disease, a theory that has been discredited.) Roast for 30–40 minutes in the oven, until crispy. Shake the pan about halfway through cooking to ensure even roasting. Let cool before serving.

Makes 4–6 servings.

This simple recipe lends itself to creative variations!

Spicy Roasted Edamame

Substitute edamame for the chickpeas for an equally satisfying treat.

Spicy Roasted Nuts

Substitute a blend or a single variety of nut, such as almonds, cashews, peanuts, or walnuts. The nuts will only need to roast for 15–20 minutes, or until fragrant.

Cooking Dry Beans

You can use canned beans in this recipe as a time-saver, but you will get better results if you prepare your own. These methods work for any type of dry beans, except for lentils, which do not need to be precooked. Here are two methods, the foolproof, slower method for cooking tender beans, and a quick method for when you are in a hurry.

Hot-Soak Method

Place the beans in a pot and add 10 cups of water for every 2 cups of beans. Heat to boiling and boil for an additional 2–3 minutes. Remove the beans from the heat, cover, and let stand for 4–24 hours. Drain the beans, discard the soaking water, and rinse with fresh, cool water. Use immediately.

Quick-Soak Method

Place the beans in a large pot and add 10 cups of water for every 2 cups of beans.

(continued)

Bring to a boil and boil for an additional 2–3 minutes.

Drain the beans, discard the soaking water, and rinse with fresh, cool water.

For more information, recipes, and techniques for cooking beans, see http://www.usdrybeans.com/recipes.

Hummus

If you have been buying hummus at the store, you will not believe how easy it is to prepare at home. You could add some roasted red pepper (minus the skin and seeds) or roasted garlic for extra flavor. The possibilities are really endless.

2 cups canned garbanzo beans, or cooked from dry (page 139)
¼ cup water
1 clove garlic, peeled
2 tablespoons extra virgin olive oil
2 tablespoons lemon juice
1 tablespoon sesame seeds (optional)
Dash freshly ground black pepper
Paprika for garnish (optional)

Blend all the ingredients except the paprika in a food processor until smooth. Garnish with paprika, if desired.

Makes 6–8 servings.

Baked Kale Chips

1 bunch of kale (6–8 ounces), trimmed, ribs removed, cut into
    pieces, washed and spun dry
2 tablespoons extra virgin olive oil
Sea salt to taste

Make sure the kale is completely dry before making this recipe.

Preheat the oven to 300°F. Mix the kale, olive oil, and sea salt well. Spread the kale on a cookie sheet and bake for about 20 minutes. Let cool before serving.

Makes 8 servings.

Roasted Cauliflower "Popcorn"

1 large head of cauliflower—about 2 pounds, cut into small chunks
2 tablespoons extra virgin olive oil
¼–½ teaspoon sea salt
¼–½ teaspoon chili powder
⅛ teaspoon garlic powder

Preheat the oven to 450°F. Line a cookie sheet with nonstick aluminum foil. Place the cauliflower in a bowl and toss with the olive oil and seasonings. (I don't normally use garlic powder, but it is the best way to truly mix the flavors.) Bake for 40–45 minutes. Cool and serve.

Makes 8–10 servings.

Salt-Free Pickles

1½ cups apple cider vinegar
1 tablespoon sugar
¼ cup water
2 tablespoons pickling spice
4–5 small cucumbers (pickle-sized)
2 to 3 cloves garlic, thinly sliced

Place the vinegar, sugar, water, and pickling spice in a saucepan. Bring to a boil and boil for 3 minutes. Let cool. Place the cucumbers and garlic in a glass bowl that can be covered.

Pour the liquid over the cucumbers and garlic and cover. Make sure the cucumbers are completely covered by the vinegar mixture. Keep refrigerated for 3 days, mixing once a day. After 3 days, the pickles are ready to eat. Do not keep for more than 2 weeks. Because these pickles are salt-free, they are not preserved like conventional pickles.

Nonfat Fruit-Flavored Yogurt

Everyone loves yogurt, but they don't always like the artificial sweeteners in light yogurts. The solution is to create your own! The simple way to make a fruit yogurt is to mix 2 tablespoons of no-added-sugar jam or preserves into 6 fluid ounces of plain nonfat yogurt. Strawberry, raspberry, orange, peach, and more—it's so easy. Or make vanilla yogurt by adding ½ teaspoon vanilla extract. Add some lime or lemon juice for citrusy flavor.

Dinner

Simple Baked Salmon

  6 salmon filets (about 4 ounces each)
  3 tablespoons fresh lime juice
  3 tablespoons honey
  2 tablespoons extra virgin olive oil
  1 lemon, cut into wedges

Place the salmon filets in a glass or ceramic baking dish, about 9 by 13 inches long. Combine the lime juice, honey, and olive oil in a small bowl and stir to create a marinade. Brush the marinade over the salmon. Refrigerate, covered, for 30 minutes. Preheat the oven to 400°F and set a rack in the middle of the oven. Bake for 15 minutes, or until cooked through. Serve immediately with lemon wedges. (You can also refrigerate the leftovers for use in a lunchtime salad.)

Makes 6 servings.

Baked Tilapia

You can use tilapia filets in place of the salmon. Marinate for no more than 15 minutes. Bake in a 375°F oven for 10–12 minutes, or until the fish flakes easily with a fork. To make the tilapia more flavorful, serve it topped with one of my salsas, such as Peach Salsa (page 185) or Mango Tango Black Bean Salsa (page 187).

You can make this recipe with most types of fish filets.

Faux Pasta e Fagioli alla Venezia

¼ cup extra virgin olive oil
1 cup onions, chopped coarse
1 cup carrots, chopped coarse
1 celery stalk with leaves, chopped coarse
1 tablespoon garlic, chopped fine
1 cup reduced-sodium chicken broth or Homemade Vegetable
  Broth (page 133), or water
1 can (14 ounces) kidney beans, or 2 cups cooked from dry
  (page 139)
3 plum tomatoes, chopped
1 teaspoon dried rosemary, crushed
¼ teaspoon crushed red pepper flakes
¼ teaspoon dried sage
4 cups shredded zucchini (page 144)
3 tablespoons fresh basil, chopped fine, or 1 teaspoon dried
Freshly ground black pepper
About ½ cup Parmesan, as desired, for garnish

Heat the oil in a large heavy saucepan over medium-high heat. Add the onions and sauté until they begin to turn golden. Add the carrots, celery, and garlic. Cook for a few minutes more, stirring occasionally.

In a medium-sized pot, heat the broth or water to boiling. Add the beans, tomatoes, sautéed vegetables, rosemary, red pepper flakes, and sage. Turn the heat to high and bring to a boil. Reduce the heat to a simmer. Cook, covered, until the beans are tender, about 15 minutes.

Transfer about 2 ladlefuls of beans and their liquid to a food processor and process to a thick purée, then stir back into the soup.

About 2 minutes before serving, bring the soup to a boil and add the zucchini. Stir occasionally while the zucchini cooks, about 2 minutes. Remove from the heat and stir in the basil and pepper to taste. Ladle into soup bowls and sprinkle each serving with Parmesan.

Makes 6 servings.

Recipe adapted from the Michigan Bean Commission.

Spiral Cuts

For an easy way to shred your zucchini, there are inexpensive tools that create spiral cuts of vegetables such as squash or carrots. Spiral-cut zucchini makes a great lower-calorie substitute for pasta, and is much faster to prepare than spaghetti squash.

Garbanzo Bean Curry with Potatoes

6 tablespoons extra virgin olive oil
2 medium onions, thinly sliced
1 teaspoon finely chopped fresh gingerroot
1 teaspoon cumin
1 teaspoon coriander
1 clove garlic, minced
1 teaspoon chili powder
2 small (or 1 medium) jalapeño peppers, seeds and ribs removed, finely diced

¼ cup fresh cilantro leaves
⅔ cup water
1 large Idaho potato, peeled and cut into ½-inch cubes
1 can (14 ounces) garbanzo beans, drained, or 2 cups cooked
    from dry (page 139)
1 tablespoon fresh lemon juice

Heat the oil in a large saucepan over medium heat. Add the onions and sauté until golden brown, about 20 minutes. Reduce the heat, add the gingerroot, cumin, coriander, garlic, chili powder, jalapeños, and cilantro, and stir-fry for 2 minutes. Add the water to the pan and stir well to mix.

Add the potato and the garbanzo beans to the mixture, cover, and simmer, stirring occasionally, for 5–7 minutes, or until the potato cubes are soft. Sprinkle the lemon juice over the curry mixture. Serve immediately.

Makes 4 servings.

Recipe adapted from *What's Cooking Indian*, by Shehzad Husain. ThunderBay Press, 1997.

Risotto with Lentils, Mushrooms, Leeks, and Pine Nuts

2 tablespoons pine nuts
1 pound white mushrooms
½ pound (2 small) leeks
4 cups Homemade Vegetable Broth (page 133), or reduced-
    sodium beef or chicken broth
⅓ cup red wine vinegar
2 teaspoons dried rosemary, crushed, or 2 tablespoons fresh
⅛ teaspoon salt
Dash freshly ground black pepper
1 tablespoon extra virgin olive oil
2 cloves garlic, minced
1 cup arborio rice

Place the pine nuts in a single layer in a dry heavy-bottomed skillet and toast over medium-high heat for several minutes. Stir or shake the pan frequently, until the nuts are lightly browned and emit a roasted scent. Set aside.

Brush the mushrooms clean, rinse, and cut into thick slices. Set aside.

Trim off the root ends and dark-green portions of the leeks. Cut the leeks in half lengthwise and rinse well under water to remove any grit. Slice crosswise into thin half-rounds. Set aside.

Bring the broth to a simmer, turn off the heat, and keep handy in a warm spot on the stove. In a stainless steel, enameled, or cast-iron skillet, combine the mushrooms, leeks, vinegar, rosemary, salt, and pepper. Bring to a simmer over medium-high heat, reduce the heat to low, and sauté, stirring frequently, about 10 minutes, until the mushrooms have released their liquid and most of it has evaporated. Do not overcook, or the mushrooms will turn rubbery.

In a large, heavy-bottomed saucepan, heat the olive oil over medium heat.

Stir in the garlic, add the rice, and sauté for about a minute.

Add the broth ½ cup at a time, stirring almost constantly and waiting until the liquid is absorbed before each addition. The rice will take about 25 minutes to cook.

When the last addition of broth has been absorbed and the rice is tender, transfer it to a warmed serving bowl, stir in the mushroom mixture and the pine nuts, and serve hot.

Makes 4–6 servings.

Penne with Tomato Sauce

2 tablespoons extra virgin olive oil
3 large garlic cloves, minced
2 medium onions, thinly sliced

4 pounds flavorful tomatoes, chopped
1 teaspoon dried thyme, or 1 tablespoon fresh
½ teaspoon crushed dried rosemary, or 1 teaspoon fresh
1 tablespoon crushed dried basil, or 2 tablespoons fresh
Dash salt
Dash freshly ground black pepper
1 pound (dry) penne pasta, cooked according to the package
   directions

Heat the oil in a large saucepan over medium heat.

Add the garlic and onions, stir, and sauté for 8 minutes. Reduce the heat as needed to prevent browning.

Add the tomatoes, thyme, and rosemary to the saucepan and bring to a boil over medium heat, stirring occasionally. Reduce the heat and simmer for 45 minutes. Add the basil and simmer another 5 minutes. Season with salt and pepper. Top the penne with the tomato sauce.

Makes 6–8 servings.

Bulgur Salad with Poblanos

2 cups water
1 cup bulgur (cracked wheat)
1 large ripe but firm tomato
2 tablespoons extra virgin olive oil
1 medium-sized poblano pepper, cored, seeded, and finely
   chopped
¼ cup coarsely chopped fresh basil
1 coarsely chopped scallion (green onion)
Juice of ½ large lime
Dash salt
Freshly ground black pepper

In a saucepan, bring the water to a boil over high heat.

Add the bulgur, stir once, and reduce the heat to a simmer. Simmer until most of the water has been absorbed and the wheat begins to seethe, about 6 minutes.

Remove from the heat, cover, and set aside for 15 minutes. The bulgur will absorb the rest of the water and become tender.

Meanwhile, fill a separate small saucepan about 3 inches deep with water; heat to boiling. Cut an X on the bottom of the tomato. Drop the tomato into the hot water for 30–60 seconds. Remove with a slotted spoon. Peel off the skin. Cut the tomato in half around the middle and squeeze to remove the seeds. Then cut into ½-inch dice. (This is called tomato concassé.)

Put the bulgur in a large strainer or colander and cool under running cold water. Shake and gently press out all the excess water. Dump into a large bowl.

With a large fork, stir in the oil to help keep the grains separated, then add the poblano, basil, scallion, tomato, and lime juice. Season with a little salt and pepper.

Makes 6 servings.

Rice with Black-Eyed Peas, Lentils, and Tomatoes

Extra virgin olive oil, in a pump mister
1 large onion, peeled and finely chopped
1 garlic clove, peeled and minced
3 cups water
¾ cup long-grain white rice
¾ cup lentils
1 can (16 ounces) black-eyed peas, drained, or 2 cups cooked from dry (page 139)
1 can (28 ounces) low-sodium diced tomatoes
1½ tablespoons chili powder

½ teaspoon cumin
1 teaspoon crushed dried oregano
¼ teaspoon cayenne pepper
Dash salt
Dash freshly ground black pepper

Spray the bottom of a large nonstick sauté pan with olive oil.

Add the onion and garlic and spray again, so that everything is lightly coated with oil. Set over medium heat and sauté until translucent, about 5 minutes, reducing the heat to prevent browning.

Scrape into a large pot, add the remaining ingredients, except for the salt and pepper, and bring to a boil over medium-high heat, stirring occasionally. Reduce the heat and simmer, partially covered, until the rice is tender, about 30 minutes, stirring occasionally to ensure that everything is evenly distributed. Season with salt and pepper to taste.

Makes 8 servings.

Barley with Wild Rice

3–3½ cups reduced-sodium chicken broth or Homemade
    Vegetable Broth (page 133)
½ cup medium pearl barley (not quick-cooking)
⅓ cup wild rice
1 small onion, peeled and finely chopped
Extra virgin olive oil, in a pump mister
Freshly ground black pepper

In a large saucepan, bring the broth to a boil, stir in the barley and wild rice, cover, and reduce the heat. Simmer, stirring every 10 or 15 minutes, until the grains are tender and the broth is absorbed, about 40 minutes total. If the grains still seem chewy, add more broth and cook for 5–10 minutes longer.

Meanwhile, place the chopped onion in a sauté pan and spray with just enough olive oil so that all the onion pieces are very lightly coated.

Sauté over medium-high heat until the onion just starts to brown, about 12 minutes. Set aside.

When the barley and wild rice are cooked, stir in the onion, taste, and season with pepper.

Serve immediately.

Makes 4 servings.

Whole Wheat Couscous with Mushrooms

2½ cups reduced-sodium beef or chicken broth, or Homemade
    Vegetable Broth (page 133)
3 tablespoons coarsely chopped sun-dried tomatoes
6 ounces small fresh mushrooms
1 clove garlic, minced
1½ cups whole wheat couscous
½ cup chopped black olives
3 tablespoons chopped fresh Italian parsley
Salt and freshly ground black pepper

In a large shallow pot, bring the broth and tomatoes to a boil. Wash the mushrooms, trimming the stem ends but leaving the stems in place. (If large, cut into pieces.) Add the mushrooms and garlic to the broth and simmer until just tender, about 3 minutes. Stir in the couscous, cover, remove from the heat, and set aside for 5 minutes. Stir in the olives and parsley. Taste and season with a little salt, if necessary, and pepper.

Serve immediately.

Makes 4 servings.

Barley Risotto with Butternut Squash and Kale

5 cups water
½ pound kale
5½ cups reduced-sodium chicken broth or Homemade Vegetable
  Broth (page 133)
1 tablespoon extra virgin olive oil
1 large onion, chopped
1½ cups pearl barley (not quick-cooking), rinsed
½ cup red wine vinegar
¾ pound butternut squash, peeled and cut into ¾-inch cubes
Salt and freshly ground black pepper
¼ cup fresh grated Parmesan, to garnish

Bring 4 cups of the water to boil in a large pot. With a sharp knife, remove the stems and thick ribs from the kale leaves and add to the water. Boil the leaves until tender, about 5 minutes.

Drain. When cool enough to handle, squeeze out the excess water, coarsely chop, and set aside.

In a medium saucepan, heat the broth and the remaining 1 cup water over medium heat until simmering. Keep warm.

In a large saucepan, heat the oil over medium heat. Add the onion and cook, stirring, until browned, about 7 minutes.

Add the barley and cook, stirring, for 1 minute. Add the vinegar and cook, stirring constantly, until it evaporates.

Add ½ cup broth and stir until most of the liquid has been absorbed.

After 5 minutes, add the squash. Continue stirring and adding broth, ½ cup at a time, as needed, until the barley is tender and creamy yet still firm, 40–50 minutes.

Stir in the reserved kale and cook, stirring constantly, until heated through, about 1 minute.

Remove from the heat and season with salt and pepper to taste. Serve garnished with Parmesan to taste.

Makes 6–8 servings.

Pesto Pizza

This is a single-serving pizza, but you could always scale up.

¼ cup Pesto (page 183)
1 whole wheat pita (or corn tortilla if you have a wheat sensitivity)
2 ounces reduced-fat mozzarella cheese, shredded
1 medium flavorful tomato, thinly sliced
1 basil leaf, thinly sliced or chopped

Preheat the oven to 400°F.

Spread the pesto on the pita. Top with the cheese, tomato, and basil. Bake for 15 minutes, or until the cheese is thoroughly melted and the edges are lightly browned.

Makes 1 serving.

Zucchini Lasagna

This recipe is especially great for using up end-of-summer veggies. An easy way to cut the basil is to roll up several leaves (stem edges inside) and then make very thin slices, called a chiffonade.

1 tablespoon extra virgin olive oil
2 large zucchinis, sliced about ¼ inch thick
4 large tomatoes, sliced about ¼ inch thick
2 medium onions, sliced very thin
1 sprig fresh basil (6–8 leaves), chopped or thinly sliced
Italian seasonings

Freshly ground black pepper
8 ounces shredded 2 percent mozzarella

Preheat the oven to 400°F.

Into a 2½-quart oval bakeware dish (such as Corningware), pour the olive oil (or spray the dish with extra virgin olive oil cooking spray). Cover the bottom of the dish with half the sliced zucchini. Layer with half of the tomatoes and then with half of the onions. Top with half of the sliced basil, Italian seasonings (or other herbs from your garden), and black pepper to taste. Then add a layer of about half the shredded cheese. Repeat with another layer of zucchini, tomatoes, onions, seasonings, and cheese.

Bake about 30 minutes, uncovered. Let cool for 5 minutes before serving.

Makes 6 servings.

Creamy Rice with Fresh Peas

3 cans (14 fluid ounces each) reduced-sodium chicken broth or about 5 cups Homemade Vegetable Broth (page 133)
1 tablespoon vegetable oil
1 small onion, peeled and finely chopped
1 garlic clove, peeled and finely chopped
¾ cup arborio rice
1 pound fresh peas, shelled, to make about 1 cup (or use frozen peas)

In a saucepan or large pot, heat the broth to boiling.

Meanwhile, place a large saucepan over medium heat. Add the vegetable oil.

When the oil is hot, add the onion and cook for 6 minutes, reducing the heat so the onions do not brown. Add the garlic and sauté until just golden brown. (If the garlic gets too dark, it will be bitter.)

Stir the rice into the onions and cook until the rice changes from its vaguely translucent color to an opaque white.

Add ½ cup of broth to the rice and stir until most of the liquid has been absorbed. Continue stirring and adding broth until the rice is tender and creamy, about 22 minutes. Some of the broth or water should not have been absorbed, leaving the rice soft and slightly soupy in texture.

While the rice is cooking, cook the peas. To steam, in a small saucepan, heat 1 inch of water to boiling. Place the peas in a steaming basket (or strainer) and cook until tender, about 2 minutes for fresh or 3 minutes for frozen.

When the rice is cooked, stir in the peas and cook for 1 minute to warm and blend the flavors.

Makes 4 servings.

Fajitas with Pico de Gallo

1 pound boneless beef top round or top sirloin steak, cut ¾ inch thick
8 flour tortillas (about 8 inches in diameter each), warmed

Marinade

2 tablespoons fresh lime juice
2 teaspoons vegetable oil
2 cloves garlic, crushed

Pico de Gallo

½ cup diced zucchini
½ cup seeded, chopped tomato
¼ cup chopped fresh cilantro
¼ cup prepared picante sauce or salsa
1 tablespoon fresh lime juice

Combine the marinade ingredients.

Place the steak in a plastic bag; add the marinade, turning to coat. Close the bag securely and marinate in the refrigerator 20–30 minutes, turning once. Remove the steak and discard the residual marinade.

Meanwhile, prepare the pico de gallo: In a medium bowl, combine the ingredients and mix well.

Place the steak on a grill pan (or broiler). Grill 12 to 16 minutes for medium-rare to medium doneness, turning once. (Or broil, 2 to 3 inches from the heat, 12 to 15 minutes.)

Trim the fat from the steak. Carve the steak crosswise into slices; serve in the tortillas with the pico de gallo.

Makes 8 servings.

Recipe adapted from the National Cattlemen's Beef Association.

Updated Beef Stroganoff

1½ cups (dry) farfalle (bow tie) pasta
1 pound beef tenderloin or beef tenderloin tips
3 tablespoons extra virgin olive oil
Freshly ground black pepper
½ pound mushrooms cut into ½-inch slices
½ cup coarsely chopped onion, or 1 small onion, chopped
¼ cup all-purpose flour
1½ cups reduced-sodium beef broth
1 tablespoon sliced green onions (scallions) for garnish

Cook the pasta according to the package directions. Drain, return to the pot, and cover to keep warm.

Trim the fat from the beef; cut into 1-by-½-inch pieces.

Heat 1 tablespoon of the olive oil in a large skillet over medium-high heat. Add the beef (half at a time) and stir-fry 1–2 minutes, or until the outside surface is no longer pink.

Remove from the skillet; place on a warm plate, season with pepper to taste, and cover to keep warm.

Using the same skillet, add the remaining 2 tablespoons olive oil and cook the mushrooms and onion 2 minutes, or until tender; stir in the flour.

Gradually add the broth, stirring until blended. Bring to a boil; cook and stir 2 minutes.

Return the beef to the skillet; heat through.

Serve the beef mixture over the pasta. Sprinkle with the scallions.

Makes 4 servings.

Recipe adapted from the National Cattlemen's Beef Association.

Quick Steak and Vegetable Soup

1 pound boneless beef top sirloin steak, cut ¾ inch thick
1 can (13½–14½ fluid ounces) reduced-sodium beef broth
1½ cups water
1 large onion, chopped
½ pound potatoes, cut into ½-inch pieces
½ pound carrots, cut into ½-inch pieces
1 cup frozen peas
¼ cup chopped assorted fresh herbs (parsley, chives, thyme, basil)
2 tablespoons balsamic vinegar
2 teaspoons vegetable oil
½ teaspoon freshly ground black pepper

Trim the fat from the steak. Cut the steak lengthwise into 3 strips and then crosswise into ½-inch-thick pieces.

In a large saucepan, combine the broth, water, onion, potatoes, carrots, and peas. Bring to a boil; reduce the heat to low.

Simmer, uncovered, 15 minutes, or until the vegetables are tender. Stir in the herbs and the vinegar.

Meanwhile, in a large nonstick skillet, heat the oil over medium-high heat until hot.

Add the beef (half at a time) and stir-fry 2–3 minutes, or until the outside surface is no longer pink. (Do not overcook.) Season with the pepper.

Divide the beef evenly among 4 individual soup bowls.

Ladle the vegetables and broth mixture over the beef. Serve immediately.

Makes 4 servings.

Recipe adapted from the National Cattlemen's Beef Association.

Stir-Fry Beef and Spinach with Noodles

1 pound beef round tip steak, cut ⅛ to ¼ inch thick
6 ounces (dry) thin spaghetti
1 package (10 ounces) fresh spinach, stems removed, thinly sliced
1 can (8 ounces) sliced water chestnuts, drained
¼ cup sliced scallions (green onions)
2 tablespoons chopped red chili peppers

Marinade
¼ cup hoisin sauce
2 tablespoons reduced-sodium soy sauce
1 tablespoon water
2 teaspoons dark sesame oil
2 large cloves garlic, crushed
¼ teaspoon crushed red pepper flakes

Stack the beef pieces and cut lengthwise in half and then crosswise into 1-inch-wide strips. Combine the marinade ingredients and pour half over the beef in a glass bowl. Cover and marinate in the refrigerator 10 minutes. Reserve the remaining marinade.

Meanwhile, cook the pasta according to the package directions; drain and return to the pan to keep warm.

Remove the beef from the marinade; discard the used marinade. Heat a large nonstick wok or skillet over medium-high heat until hot.

Add the beef (half at a time) and stir-fry 1 to 2 minutes, or until the outside surface is no longer pink. (Do not overcook.) Remove from the wok with a slotted spoon; place on a warm plate and cover to keep warm.

In the same wok or skillet, combine the pasta, spinach, water chestnuts, scallions, and reserved marinade; cook until the spinach is wilted and the mixture is heated through, stirring occasionally. Return the beef to the pan; mix lightly. Garnish with the chili peppers.

Makes 4 servings.

Recipe adapted from the National Cattlemen's Beef Association.

Super-Quick Chicken Stir-Fry

2 tablespoons canola oil or peanut oil
1 pound boneless, skinless chicken breasts, cut into ½-by-2-inch strips
1 small yellow onion, cut into ½-inch strips
8 ounces broccoli florets
8 ounces cauliflower florets
1 medium red bell pepper, seeded and cut into ½-inch strips
1 medium yellow bell pepper, seeded and cut into ½-inch strips
¼ cup low-sodium stir-fry sauce

Heat the oil in a large skillet or wok over medium-high heat. When the oil is hot (but not smoking), add half of the chicken strips and stir-fry, using a wooden spatula, 1–2 minutes, until browned on all sides.

Remove the chicken, place on warm plate, and repeat with the rest of the chicken. Cover the plate with a pot lid or aluminum foil to keep warm.

Add additional oil to the pan, if needed. Add the onion and sauté 2–3 minutes; add the broccoli, cauliflower, and peppers and stir-fry an additional 3–4 minutes, until crisp-tender.

Add the stir-fry sauce, return the chicken to the pan, and stir well to reheat the chicken and combine all the ingredients.

Makes 4 servings.

Peach and Balsamic Glazed Pork Chops

1 can (10 ounces) peach slices in extra-light syrup, drained (or 2 medium peaches, peeled and sliced ¾ inch thick)
2 tablespoons peach preserves
¼ cup water
¼ cup balsamic vinegar
1 tablespoon extra virgin olive oil
4 boneless pork loin chops (4 ounces each), ¾ inch thick
1 teaspoon freshly ground black pepper

Combine the peaches, preserves, water, and balsamic vinegar in a medium bowl.

Heat olive oil in a large skillet over medium-high heat until hot. Season the chops with pepper. Add the chops to the skillet; brown well on both sides.

Add the peach mixture to the skillet; reduce the heat to low. Cover; cook 5 minutes.

Serve the chops with the peach mixture.

Makes 4 servings.

Carnitas

Traditionally, carnitas are made from pork butt or shoulder, which you could certainly do. However, I personally did not appreciate the anatomy lesson that I found in my pot when using these cuts. So I use a roast, which already has everything removed but the meat.

3 pounds pork roast
3 cups orange juice
2 cups beef broth or Homemade Vegetable Broth (page 133),
   to cover meat
5 cloves garlic, peeled and smashed
1 bay leaf
1 onion, peeled and quartered

In a large pot, brown the pork on both sides. Add in the orange juice, then add broth to cover meat. Add garlic, bay leaf, and onion. Bring the liquid to a boil, then turn it down to a simmer for 2½–3 hours. Near the end of cooking, test tenderness with a fork. The meat should be very tender.

At the end of the cooking time, turn up the heat briefly to help evaporate excess liquid.

At this point there are two ways to prepare the carnitas. First, cut into 1-inch chunks. Then either transfer to a pan and gently sauté to slightly crisp the meat, or shred the chunks with two forks, much like preparing pulled pork.

Serve on top of salad greens topped with Citrus Vinaigrette (page 182), my lighter preference, or with whole grain tortillas.

Makes about 8 servings.

Skillet BBQ'd Chicken

2 tablespoons extra virgin olive oil
1 tablespoon red wine vinegar
¼ cup BBQ sauce (or make your own with 2 tablespoons ketchup, 2 tablespoons orange juice, and 1 teaspoon hot sauce)
1 teaspoon chili powder
4 boneless, skinless chicken breasts (4 ounces each)
1 teaspoon dried oregano
1 teaspoon dried basil
½ teaspoon chopped fresh Italian parsley

Blend the oil, vinegar, BBQ sauce, and chili powder in a shallow glass dish. Add the chicken and turn to coat. Cover and marinate 30 minutes in the refrigerator.

Heat a nonstick skillet over medium-high heat until hot. Drain the chicken, reserving the marinade. Brown both sides of the chicken and add the reserved marinade.

Bring to a boil. Cover, reduce the heat to low, and simmer for 10 minutes. Add the oregano, basil, and parsley, mix into the sauce, and cook an additional 2 minutes.

Makes 4 servings.

Kung Pao Chicken

1½ pounds boneless, skinless chicken breasts, cut into 1-inch cubes
3 teaspoons low-sodium soy sauce
½ cup rice wine vinegar
2 teaspoons sesame oil
2 tablespoons peanut oil
1 clove garlic, minced
1 tablespoon cayenne pepper
1 medium carrot, sliced diagonally into ¼-inch slices
½ cup cashews
1 medium zucchini, julienned or cut with a vegetable spiral
  cutter (page 144)
2 scallions (green onions), cut into ¼-inch slices

Marinate the chicken in 2 teaspoons of the soy sauce, 2 tablespoons of the rice wine vinegar, and the sesame oil in a covered glass bowl, refrigerated, for at least 30 minutes.

Heat a large skillet or wok over medium-high heat, then add the peanut oil. Add the chicken and stir-fry until browned on all sides. Remove the chicken and place on a warm plate, covered.

Lower the heat to medium, add additional peanut oil to the pan if needed, and sauté the garlic and cayenne pepper for about 2 minutes. Return the heat to medium-high, add the carrot slices and chicken, and stir-fry another 2 minutes.

Add the remaining vinegar and soy sauce, the cashews, and the zucchini. Bring to a rapid boil and stir in the scallions. Serve immediately.

Makes 4–6 servings.

Kung Pao Tofu

You can substitute tofu for the chicken to make this into a vegetarian meal.

Jerk Pork

4 boneless pork loin chops (4 ounces each), ¾ inch thick
1 tablespoon extra virgin olive oil
Freshly ground black pepper

Marinade

½ teaspoon allspice
½ teaspoon salt
1 tablespoon freshly ground black pepper
1 clove garlic, minced
1 scallion (green onion), thinly sliced
1½ tablespoons Worcestershire sauce
1 medium jalapeño pepper, seeds and ribs removed, finely diced
¼ cup olive oil

Combine the marinade ingredients and pour over the pork chops in a glass bowl. Let stand in the refrigerator, covered, for 12 hours.

Heat olive oil in a large skillet over medium-high heat until hot. Season the chops with pepper. Add the chops to the skillet; brown well on both sides. Reduce heat to medium, cover, and cook 5 minutes.

Makes 4 servings.

Halibut with Salted Black Beans and Chilies

1 pound halibut steak
1 teaspoon salt
1 teaspoon finely chopped fresh gingerroot
¼ teaspoon freshly ground white pepper
4 scallions (green onions)
2 medium jalapeño peppers, seeds and ribs removed
3 tablespoons vegetable oil
1 tablespoon water
1 cup canned black beans, drained, or cooked from dry (page 139)
2 teaspoons finely chopped garlic
1 cup reduced-sodium chicken broth or Homemade Vegetable
   Broth (page 133)
Spinach or lettuce leaves

Rinse the fish and pat it dry. Mix the salt, gingerroot, and white pepper. Coat both sides of the fish with the mixture and place in a glass casserole. Cover and refrigerate 30 minutes.

Cut 3 scallions diagonally into 1-inch pieces. Cut the remaining scallion into thin slices.

Cut the jalapeños into very thin slices.

Heat a wok or medium skillet over medium heat until hot. Add 2 tablespoons of the vegetable oil and tilt to coat the bottom and sides.

Sauté the fish 2 minutes, or until brown, turning once. Reduce the heat to low, add the water, cover, and simmer 10 minutes, turning after 3 minutes. Remove the fish from the pan.

Heat the pan until medium hot. Add the remaining 1 tablespoon vegetable oil.

Add the beans, jalapeños, garlic, and scallion pieces. Stir-fry 1 minute. Add the broth and heat to boiling.

Add the fish, turning to coat with the sauce. Heat 2 minutes.

Line a serving platter with spinach or lettuce leaves. Place the fish on the leaves and sprinkle with the scallion slices.

Makes 4 servings.

Lemon Chicken Breasts

4 boneless, skinless chicken breasts (4 ounces each)
½ cup cornmeal
1 teaspoon lemon pepper seasoning mix
1 tablespoon extra virgin olive oil
1 tablespoon butter
¼ cup lemon juice

Wash and dry the chicken breasts.

Put the cornmeal on a plate, add the lemon pepper, and mix.

Drop the chicken on the cornmeal, then flip to cover both sides with the meal.

Heat the olive oil over medium heat in a skillet.

Add the chicken. Cook the first side until light color comes about halfway up the side of the chicken. Flip and cook the other side. The chicken surface should be light to dark brown. (Cut into one of the thicker pieces if you're unsure about doneness.)

When the chicken looks done, add the butter and lemon juice. Stir with a wooden spoon to loosen all the crusty browned pieces in the bottom of the skillet.

Place the chicken on plates and cover each with some of the sauce.

Makes 4 servings.

Caribbean Chicken

2–3 whole boneless, skinless chicken breasts, 1–1½ pounds
1 teaspoon salt
Dash freshly ground black pepper
Dash paprika
Dash ground cayenne pepper
1 tablespoon extra virgin olive oil
½ medium onion, thinly sliced
1 clove garlic, minced
½ cup water
1 teaspoon ground ginger
2 oranges, to yield:
    2 teaspoons grated orange peel
    1 cup fresh orange juice
    Slices of 1 orange, peeled
2 cups fresh pineapple, cut into chunks

Sprinkle the chicken with the salt, pepper, paprika, and cayenne pepper. Heat the oil in large skillet over medium-high heat. Add the chicken and onion and sauté until well browned on all sides. Lower the heat to medium, add the garlic, and sauté for 2 minutes.

Combine the water, ginger, orange peel, and orange juice. Pour over the chicken. Cover, lower the heat to medium-low, and simmer 40 minutes, or until tender. Remove the chicken to a warm serving platter.

Add the pineapple chunks and orange slices to the pan drippings and heat to boiling, stirring. Add the chicken and heat for 2 minutes, spooning the fruit mixture over the chicken. Serve immediately.

Makes 4 servings.

Vegetarian Chili

2 cans (14½ ounces each) low-sodium diced tomatoes or 2 pounds
  fresh, flavorful tomatoes, peeled and cut into chunks
1 can (15 ounces) black beans, drained and rinsed, or 2 cups
  cooked from dry (page 139)
1 can (15 ounces) kidney beans, drained and rinsed, or 2 cups
  cooked from dry (page 139)
2 cups water
2 tablespoons chili powder
2 tablespoons paprika
1 teaspoon freshly ground black pepper
1 package frozen sweet corn (or fresh, cut off 2 large ears)
½ cup broccoli florets
½ cup cauliflower florets
½ cup carrots, sliced into 1-inch chunks
1 medium onion, diced
1 medium red bell pepper, seeded and sliced into ½-inch strips
¼ cup shredded reduced-fat cheddar cheese (optional)

In a large pot over medium heat, cook the tomatoes, beans, water, and seasonings 15 minutes.

Add the vegetables and reduce the heat to maintain a simmer (low to medium-low). Cook 15–30 minutes. (You can add any other vegetables you think would be interesting.)

If the chili starts to get really thick, add extra water. Serve garnished with cheese, as desired.

Makes 10 servings.

To remove the skin from whole tomatoes, heat a medium pot of water to boiling. Cut an X into the bottom of each tomato. Use a slotted spoon to dunk the tomatoes into the boiling water. Keep in the water for 30–60 seconds, until the skin begins to curl back slightly at the X mark. Remove with the slotted spoon and peel off the skin.

South of the Border Tofu Enchiladas

1 tablespoon extra virgin olive oil
½ cup chopped onion (about 1 small yellow onion)
¾ cup chopped green bell pepper
1 can (4 ounces) chopped mild green chilies
1 clove garlic, minced
½ teaspoon whole cumin seeds
1 teaspoon fresh cilantro, minced
12 ounces firm silken tofu, drained and mashed
3 medium flavorful tomatoes, diced (or 14½-ounce can low-sodium diced tomatoes)
8 whole wheat tortillas (8 inches each)
Hot Black Bean Salsa with Tomatoes and Cilantro (page 187)
½ cup low-fat cheddar cheese, shredded

Preheat the oven to 350°F.

Use a small piece of waxed paper to spread the olive oil onto the bottom and sides of a 9-by-13-inch baking dish.

In a large bowl, combine all the ingredients except the tortillas, salsa, and cheese.

Place ½ cup of the mixture in the center of each tortilla and roll.

Place the enchiladas in the baking dish, seam side down. Pour the salsa over the enchiladas. Sprinkle with the shredded cheese.

Cover the baking dish with aluminum foil and bake for 25–30 minutes.

Makes 8 servings.

Steak and Roasted Vegetable Salad

Salad

1 medium zucchini, cut diagonally into 1-inch pieces
1 medium yellow crookneck squash, cut diagonally into 1-inch pieces
2 cups frozen sliced onion and pepper mix
16 small mushrooms
1 tablespoon extra virgin olive oil
1 pound boneless beef top sirloin steak, cut 1 inch thick
8 cups romaine, cut into 1-inch strips

Seasoning

¼ cup extra virgin olive oil
2 tablespoons balsamic vinegar
2 large cloves garlic, minced
1 teaspoon dried rosemary leaves, crushed
¼ teaspoon freshly ground black pepper

Dressing

¼ cup extra virgin olive oil
¼ cup red wine vinegar
1 teaspoon dried oregano
1 teaspoon chopped fresh Italian parsley
Dash freshly ground black pepper

Preheat the oven to 425°F. Place the zucchini, squash, onions, peppers, and mushrooms on a cookie sheet with raised sides and drizzle with the olive oil. Combine the seasoning ingredients and drizzle over the vegetables. Roast 30–35 minutes, or until tender, stirring once.

Meanwhile, heat a large nonstick skillet over medium heat until hot. Place the beef in the skillet and cook 12–15 minutes for medium-rare to medium doneness. Turn once during cooking. Let stand 10 minutes.

Combine the dressing ingredients.

Trim the fat from the beef; carve crosswise into thin slices.

To serve, place equal amounts of romaine on each of 4 dinner plates. Arrange the beef and roasted vegetables over the lettuce. Serve immediately with the dressing.

Makes 4 servings.

Pasta and Broccoli

1 pound broccoli
2 quarts water
1½ teaspoons extra virgin olive oil
1 medium onion, thinly sliced
1 clove garlic, minced
¼ cup red wine vinegar or cooking wine
1 tablespoon chopped fresh basil (or 1 teaspoon dried)
⅛ teaspoon cayenne pepper
1 can (16 fluid ounces) tomato sauce
1 can (14 ounces) low-sodium diced tomatoes, or 3 medium flavorful tomatoes, diced
2 tablespoons golden raisins, soaked in warm water about 10–15 minutes
2 tablespoons pine nuts
Freshly ground black pepper
6 ounces dry pasta (penne or ziti)
3 tablespoons freshly grated Romano

Cut the stalks off the broccoli and separate the tops into small florets. (Note: The stalks are not used in this recipe, but you could slaw them and refrigerate to use on salads and in other meals.)

In a large saucepan, bring the water to a boil; add the broccoli florets. Cook until tender, about 5 minutes. With a slotted spoon, scoop out the broccoli and set aside. Save the cooking water.

In a large heavy-bottomed skillet, heat the oil over medium heat. Add the onion and sauté 5–10 minutes, until softened. Add the garlic and sauté until lightly browned, about 2 minutes. Add the vinegar or wine, basil, and cayenne and cook, stirring, for about 30 seconds.

Add the tomato sauce and diced tomatoes and cook, stirring, for 2 minutes. Add the broccoli and mash lightly with a wooden spoon. Reduce the heat and simmer for about 10 minutes, stirring occasionally. The sauce should have the consistency of a lumpy pea soup. Thin with a little of the cooking water, if necessary.

Drain the raisins and add them to the sauce along with the pine nuts. Season the sauce with pepper to taste and keep warm over low heat.

Reheat the broccoli-cooking water to a boil and add the pasta. Cook until al dente, 6–8 minutes. Drain. Stir the pasta into the sauce and cook for 1 or 2 minutes.

Serve with a sprinkling of the cheese.

Makes 4 servings.

Tomato Pasta Primavera

½ cup chopped onion
2 medium garlic cloves, minced
2 tablespoons extra virgin olive oil
2 cans (14½ ounces each) low-sodium diced tomatoes
½ teaspoon dried basil
2 teaspoons sugar

1 cup cooking wine
½ cup carrots, sliced on the diagonal
½ cup celery, sliced on the diagonal
¼ teaspoon freshly ground black pepper
1 pound (dry) rotini
½ cup broccoli florets
½ cup chopped fresh Italian parsley
Freshly ground white pepper

Sauté the onion and garlic in the olive oil over medium heat, about 5 minutes. Add the tomatoes, basil, sugar, wine, carrots, celery, and black pepper. Simmer 20 minutes.

Cook the pasta according to the package directions.

Add the broccoli, the parsley, and white pepper to taste to the vegetable mixture. Cook 5–10 minutes, until the broccoli is just tender. Serve over the cooked pasta.

Makes 4 servings.

Yellow Split Pea Soup with Sweet Potatoes and Mustard Greens

2 tablespoons extra virgin olive oil
1 large onion, chopped
4 cloves garlic, minced
2 teaspoons ground cumin
2 cups dried yellow split peas, rinsed
5 cups water
4 cups reduced-sodium chicken broth or Homemade Vegetable
    Broth (page 133)
1 can (14½ ounces) low-sodium diced plum tomatoes, drained
1 medium sweet potato, peeled and cut into ½-inch cubes
½ pound mustard greens, ribs removed, leaves coarsely chopped
    (8 cups; or 1½ cups frozen chopped mustard greens)
Salt and freshly ground black pepper

In a large pot, heat the oil over medium heat. Add the onion and cook, stirring, until softened, 4–5 minutes. Add the garlic and cumin and cook until fragrant, about 1 minute more.

Add the split peas, water, and broth and bring to a simmer. Reduce the heat to low, cover, and simmer until the split peas have completely broken down, about 1 hour.

Add the tomatoes, sweet potato, and mustard greens. Cover and simmer, stirring occasionally, until the vegetables are tender, 25–30 minutes more. Season with salt and pepper to taste.

Makes 6 servings.

Vegetables and Salads

Roasted Brussels Sprouts with Balsamic Vinegar and Pine Nuts

1½ pounds Brussels sprouts, halved
2 tablespoons extra virgin olive oil
1 tablespoon balsamic vinegar
2 tablespoons pine nuts

Preheat the oven to 400°F. Toss the Brussels sprouts with the oil. Place in a single layer on a baking sheet. (I like to line the sheet with nonstick aluminum foil, to prevent sticking and to ease cleanup.) Roast for 30 minutes, or until soft.

Remove to a serving plate, drizzle with the balsamic vinegar, and sprinkle with the pine nuts.

Makes 4 servings.

Braised Red Cabbage

2 tablespoons extra virgin olive oil
4 cups shredded red cabbage
1 small red apple, peeled, cored, and cut into thin slices
1 medium shallot, finely sliced
1 teaspoon butter
¼ cup (packed) brown sugar
¼ cup raspberry vinegar (or red wine vinegar)
½ teaspoon salt
¼ cup water

In a medium skillet, heat the olive oil over medium heat. Add the cabbage, apple, and shallot and sauté for 5 minutes. Add the rest of the ingredients, reduce the heat, and simmer for 20 minutes.

Makes 6 servings.

Braised Radishes

2 bunches radishes (heirloom variety, if available), about 1 pound, tops and roots trimmed
1½ cups reduced-sodium chicken broth (or Homemade Vegetable Broth, page 133)
1 tablespoon extra virgin olive oil
1 large shallot, thinly sliced
1 tablespoon balsamic vinegar
Dash freshly ground black pepper
1 tablespoon butter

Place the radishes in a skillet with the broth, olive oil, shallot, vinegar, and pepper. Cover the pan and bring to a boil. Uncover the pan and reduce the heat to medium. Cook the radishes 10–12 minutes. Add the butter and cook 1 minute more.

Makes 4 servings.

Southern Corn Casserole

4 cups sweet corn, fresh or frozen
½ cup green bell pepper, seeded and diced
½ cup red bell pepper, seeded and diced
1 medium onion, diced
1 clove garlic, minced
1 medium jalapeño pepper, seeds and ribs removed,
    finely diced
½ cup reduced-fat cheddar cheese, grated
½ cup reduced-fat Monterey Jack cheese, grated
4 eggs, slightly beaten
½ cup 2 percent milk

Preheat the oven to 350°F. In a large bowl, combine the corn, green pepper, red pepper, onion, and garlic. Mix well. Add the jalapeño and cheeses. Stir in the eggs and milk. Pour the mixture into a shallow baking dish and bake for 1 hour, until the casserole is set.

Makes 10 servings.

Hearty Dinner Salad

2 large romaine hearts, cut into ¾-inch strips
3 medium flavorful tomatoes (or 20 grape tomatoes)
½ cup shredded red cabbage
½ cup grated carrots
½ cup sliced mushrooms (optional)
¼ cup pine nuts

Toss together all the ingredients and top with your choice of dressing. Additional toppings could include sliced bell peppers, garbanzo beans, chopped hard-boiled eggs, artichoke hearts, etc.

Makes 4–6 servings.

Greek Pepper Salad

1 green bell pepper, seeded and sliced
1 red bell pepper, seeded and sliced
1 yellow bell pepper, seeded and sliced
1 unpeeled cucumber, sliced
1 tablespoon olive oil
2 tablespoons lemon juice
3 tablespoons red wine vinegar
¼ teaspoon dried oregano
½ brick (4 ounces) feta cheese, crumbled

Mix the peppers and cucumber in a bowl. Add the olive oil, lemon juice, vinegar, and oregano and mix well. Cover and marinate for at least 30 minutes in the refrigerator.

Toss well before serving and top with the cheese.

Makes 4 servings.

Lentil Rice Salad

½ cup lentils, washed
1½ cups water
¾ cup quick-cooking brown rice
1 cup chopped tomato
¼ cup sliced scallions (green onions)
1 cup diced carrots
¾ cup green bell pepper, seeded and coarsely chopped
1½ cups broccoli florets
1 tablespoon dried parsley

Dressing

3 tablespoons rice wine vinegar
1 tablespoon lemon juice
½ teaspoon Dijon mustard

Add the lentils to the water in a medium saucepan and bring to a boil. Reduce the heat, cover, and simmer for 20 minutes. Drain.

Cook the rice according to the package directions.

Mix the lentils, rice, vegetables, and parsley.

Mix the dressing ingredients and pour over the salad mixture. Chill well before serving.

Makes 8 servings.

Salade Niçoise

6 ounces *haricots verts* (skinny whole French green beans)
8 small new red potatoes, cleaned
6 cups romaine, cut into 1-inch strips
4 hard-boiled eggs, peeled and quartered
1½ cups quartered cherry tomatoes
3 cans (5 ounces each) albacore tuna, packed in olive oil
Citrus Vinaigrette (page 182)

Steam the *haricots verts* for 5 minutes in a steamer set in a saucepan, over 1 inch of boiling water. Remove and rinse in cold water in a colander.

Boil the whole red potatoes for 15 minutes. Drain and rinse under cold water and cut each in half.

On each of 4 salad plates, place a bed of romaine and top with ¼ of the green beans, potatoes, eggs, tomatoes, and tuna. Top each with ¼ of the dressing.

Makes 4 servings.

Salade Niçoise with Garbanzo Beans

For an easy vegetarian variation, replace the tuna with 2 cups of garbanzo beans (canned or cooked from dry, page 139).

Mango Walnut Salad

3 cups romaine, cut into 1-inch strips
1 very ripe mango, peeled and diced
1½ cups grape tomatoes, halved
½ cup walnut pieces
Citrus Vinaigrette (page 182)

Mix the romaine, mango, tomatoes, and walnut pieces. Top with citrus vinaigrette and toss to mix well. Serve immediately.

Makes 4 servings.

New Vegetable Bean Salad

1 small can (8 ounces) garbanzo beans, drained, or 1 cup cooked from dry (page 139)
1 small can (8 ounces) kidney beans, drained, or 1 cup cooked from dry (page 139)
1 cup sliced green beans, cooked and cooled
½ cup sliced carrots
½ cup small florets of cauliflower
½ cup small florets of broccoli
¼ cup diced onion
¼ cup rice wine vinegar
1 tablespoon dried parsley, or 2 tablespoons fresh chopped Italian parsley
1 teaspoon minced garlic

Combine the garbanzo and kidney beans with the vegetables in a bowl. In a separate small bowl, mix the vinegar with the seasonings. Add to the vegetables and mix well.

Makes 6 servings.

Caprese Salad

4 ounces buffalo mozzarella, sliced ¼ inch thick
2 medium flavorful tomatoes, sliced
4 leaves basil, cut into thin strips
Extra virgin olive oil
Balsamic vinegar

Alternate slices of mozzarella and tomato on a plate. Top with strips of basil and drizzle with olive oil and balsamic vinegar.

Makes 2 servings.

Stone Fruit Salad

2 peaches, diced
3 plums, diced
2 nectarines, diced
15 cherries, pitted and chopped
Juice from 1 lime
1 tablespoon honey
4 leaves mint (minced)

Combine all ingredients, mix well to coat. Refrigerate for 30 minutes or until ready to serve.

Makes 4 servings.

Waldorf Salad

½ cup canned pineapple tidbits, or diced fresh
2 Red Delicious apples, unpeeled, cored, and diced
2 bananas, sliced
¼ cup chopped walnuts
½ cup chopped celery
1 cup grapes, halved, seeds removed (or use seedless grapes)
¼ cup light mayonnaise or plain regular Greek yogurt
4 lettuce leaves

Drain the pineapple tidbits, reserving the juice. In a medium bowl, cover the apple pieces and banana slices with the pineapple juice to prevent browning (or use lemon juice if you used fresh pineapple). Add walnuts, celery, grapes, pineapple, and mayonnaise. Stir to coat the salad evenly with the dressing. Place each serving on a lettuce leaf and serve immediately.

Makes 4 servings.

Traditional Coleslaw

4 cups shredded green cabbage
2 cups shredded red cabbage
1 carrot, shredded
⅔ cup mayonnaise
1 tablespoon red wine vinegar
1 tablespoon apple juice
2 tablespoons extra virgin olive oil
1 tablespoon sugar (optional)
½ teaspoon celery seed

Toss both types of cabbage in a large bowl with the carrot. In a separate bowl, whisk together the remaining ingredients. Pour the mixture over the cabbage-and-carrot mixture and toss to coat thoroughly. Refrigerate for at least 30 minutes.

Makes 6 servings.

Asian Coleslaw

Dressing

8 tablespoons rice vinegar
6 tablespoons extra virgin olive oil
3 tablespoons creamy natural peanut butter
3 tablespoons reduced-sodium soy sauce
2 tablespoons (packed) light brown sugar
2 tablespoons minced fresh gingerroot
2 cloves garlic, minced

Salad

5 cups thinly sliced green cabbage
2 cups thinly sliced red cabbage
1 large red bell pepper, cut into matchsticks
1 large yellow bell pepper, cut into matchsticks
4 grated carrots, or 1 cup (if you have a food processor, you
    could also process these into matchsticks for a pretty look)
½ cup cilantro, chopped (optional)

Whisk together the dressing ingredients to mix well.

Toss together the salad ingredients. Top with the dressing and toss again to mix well.

Makes 8 servings.

To make the matchstick-sized pepper strips, cut off the tops and bottoms of the peppers. Make a slice down one side of the pepper to open it up. Flatten it, place your hand on top of it, and with a very sharp butcher's knife, slice along the surface, removing the ribs and seeds. If you want to get fancy, you can also remove the skin this way. (Or not.) Then slice the pepper into matchstick-sized strips.

Farmer's Salad

Have your own garden? In late summer you are probably drowning in cucumbers and tomatoes. So make a fabulous salad!

4 medium tomatoes, cut into eighths
2 cups cucumber, cut into 1-inch chunks
Citrus Vinaigrette (page 182)

Mix the cucumbers and tomatoes and top with the dressing. As simple as that!

Makes 4 servings.

Fresh Salad Dressings

Making your own salad dressings is the only way to be sure your dressings contain healthy oils and avoid unwanted additives. And it is so easy. A side benefit is that it helps you use up your olive oil so your supply doesn't get old or develop off-flavors.

Citrus Vinaigrette

Freshly grated zest of 1 lemon
3 tablespoons fresh lemon juice
3 tablespoons water
Pinch kosher salt
Pinch freshly ground black pepper
2 tablespoons extra virgin olive oil

In a small bowl, whisk together the lemon zest and juice, water, salt, and pepper. Gradually whisk in the oil. Store refrigerated up to 3 days.

Makes 4 servings.

Dijon Vinaigrette

2 tablespoons red wine vinegar
2 tablespoons extra virgin olive oil
4 tablespoons water
1 teaspoon Dijon mustard
¼ teaspoon kosher salt
¼ teaspoon freshly ground black pepper

In a small bowl, whisk together all the ingredients. Store refrigerated up to 3 days.

Makes 4 servings.

Italian Dressing

2 tablespoons red wine vinegar
2 tablespoons extra virgin olive oil
4 tablespoons water
1 teaspoon dried oregano
1 teaspoon dried basil
¼ teaspoon dried thyme

¼ teaspoon onion powder
¼ teaspoon garlic powder
¼ teaspoon kosher salt
¼ teaspoon freshly ground black pepper

In a small bowl, whisk together all the ingredients. Store refrigerated up to 3 days.

Makes 4 servings.

Ranch Dressing

⅓ cup buttermilk
¼ cup mayonnaise
1 scallion (green onion), minced
2 tablespoons cider vinegar
½ teaspoon celery seed
¼ teaspoon freshly ground black pepper

In a small bowl, whisk together all the ingredients. Store refrigerated up to 3 days.

Makes 4 servings.

Sauces and Salsas

Pesto

2 cups fresh basil leaves, packed tightly (remove stems and discard any dried or browned edges)
⅓ cup pine nuts
3 medium cloves garlic, chopped
½ cup freshly grated Parmigiano-Reggiano
½ cup extra virgin olive oil
¼ teaspoon freshly ground black pepper, or to taste

In a food processor, pulse the basil and pine nuts for 10 seconds. Add the garlic and cheese and pulse several times.

Slowly add the olive oil in a constant stream while the food processor is on. Stop as needed to scrape down the sides with a rubber spatula. Season with pepper to taste. Store refrigerated up to 3 days.

Makes 1 cup.

Guacamole

Everyone has his or her own favorite guacamole. You can use this recipe as a starting point, then add your own embellishments. Add more peppers, add diced tomatoes, it is up to you how interesting you want to make your guac.

2 avocados
1 small onion, finely diced
1 clove garlic, peeled and minced
1 small jalapeño, seeded and ribs removed, finely chopped
Juice from 1 lime
2 tablespoons cilantro, minced (optional)

Peel and gently mash avocados in a medium serving bowl. Stir in onion, garlic, jalapeño, lime juice, and optional cilantro. Eat fresh or cover and chill for at least 30 minutes before serving.

Makes about 4 servings.

Unsweetened Applesauce

4 medium golden delicious apples
½ teaspoon cinnamon

Wash, peel, and quarter the apples. Remove all traces of the core.

Place the apples in a 1-quart saucepan and add just enough water to cover the bottom of the pan. Simmer, covered, until the apples are tender, about 10 minutes. Drain in a colander.

Press the apples through a strainer or purée in a blender. Add the cinnamon and mix well. Chill for 30 minutes before using. Store refrigerated up to 3 days.

Makes 4 servings.

Peach Salsa

3 medium ripe peaches, peeled and diced
2 medium flavorful tomatoes, peeled and diced
1 small jalapeño pepper, seeds and ribs removed, finely diced
½ medium yellow bell pepper, diced
½ small Bermuda or Vidalia onion, finely diced (freeze and save the rest for another use)
1 tablespoon chopped cilantro
1 tablespoon (packed) brown sugar
Juice of 1 lime
1 teaspoon lime zest (optional)

Combine all the ingredients in a large bowl. Mix well and refrigerate for at least 30 minutes before serving. This salsa works as a dip or as a topping for chicken, pork, or salad. Store refrigerated up to 3 days.

Makes 4 servings.

Pine Nut, Apple, Pineapple, and Grape Salsa

2 medium Granny Smith apples, cored and chopped
1 tablespoon fresh lime juice
6 slices pineapple, diced
2 cups red grapes, halved, seeds removed
½ cup toasted pine nuts
1 teaspoon (packed) brown sugar

Toss the apples with the lime juice to coat. Combine all the ingredients and chill for 30 minutes before serving. Store refrigerated up to 3 days.

Makes 4 servings.

Texas Caviar

1 can (15 ounces) black-eyed peas, or 2 cups cooked from dry (page 139)
1 can (15 ounces) garbanzo beans, or 2 cups cooked from dry (page 139)
1 cup frozen (or fresh) sweet corn
2 medium flavorful tomatoes, diced
1 medium green bell pepper, seeds and membranes removed, diced medium
1 scallion (green onion), finely chopped
1 medium jalapeño pepper, seeds and ribs removed, finely diced
2 tablespoons fresh lime juice
1 teaspoon lime zest (optional)
1 tablespoon extra virgin olive oil
½ teaspoon garlic powder
½ teaspoon ground cumin
¼ teaspoon freshly ground black pepper

Mix all the ingredients well and chill. If you are cooking the beans from dry, let them cool before adding to the mixture.

Makes 4 servings.

Three Stone Fruit Salsa

1 peach, peeled and diced
2 plums, peeled and diced
1 mango (overripe for best flavor), peeled and diced
½ cup Bermuda onion, finely diced
1 medium jalapeño pepper, seeds and ribs removed, finely diced
2 tablespoons rice vinegar

Mix all the ingredients together and refrigerate for 30 minutes. Serve as a salsa, as a topping for a salad, a side salad, or as a topping for chicken or pork. Store refrigerated up to 3 days.

Makes 4 servings.

Mango Tango Black Bean Salsa

1 can (15 ounces) black beans, rinsed and drained, or 1 cup
   cooked from dry (page 139)
1 cup frozen sweet corn, or the corn from 1 fresh cob, cooked in
   boiling water 3–4 minutes
1 medium mango, peeled, diced into ¾-inch cubes
½ small onion, finely diced (dice the whole onion and freeze half
   for later use)
2 tablespoons chopped fresh cilantro
2 tablespoons fresh lime juice
1 teaspoon garlic powder
¼ teaspoon ground cumin

In a medium bowl, combine all the ingredients. Store refrigerated up to 3 days. Serve as a dip for raw vegetables, as a side dish, or as a topping for chicken or pork.

Makes 4 servings.

Hot Black Bean Salsa with Tomatoes and Cilantro

1½ tablespoons extra virgin olive oil
1 medium onion, chopped
1 teaspoon garlic, chopped
1 pound flavorful tomatoes, coarsely chopped
1 can (15 ounces) black beans, drained and rinsed, or 2 cups
   cooked from dry (page 139)
½ teaspoon Tabasco sauce
2 tablespoons chopped fresh cilantro

Heat the oil in a small skillet over medium high-heat; add the onion and garlic. Sauté until the onion is almost translucent but still firm, about 5 minutes. Add the tomatoes and cook, stirring frequently, 2 minutes more.

Add the black beans and Tabasco and stir to combine. Cover the skillet and cook until the beans are heated through, about 2 minutes.

Remove from the heat. Stir in 1 tablespoon of the cilantro. Transfer to a serving dish and sprinkle with the remaining cilantro. Serve immediately.

This hot salsa can be a dip for vegetables or a topping for rice.

Makes 4 servings.

Adapted from the USA Dry Pea & Lentil Council.

PART III

Breakthrough Lifestyle Solutions

CHAPTER 9

Three Lifestyle Secrets to a Younger You

Figuring out how to postpone, even reverse, aging is like trying to put together a jigsaw puzzle. Piece by piece, scientists keep finding clues to fill in the picture. You've already read about how diet and nutrition are huge pieces of the puzzle. But exciting new research reveals that exercise, stress management, and quality sleeps are a big part of the picture, too. All three of these lifestyle issues have something in common: their ability to lengthen telomeres. As you know by now, the longer your telomeres, the less you age and the longer you live.

You can enjoy many more vibrant, healthy years, looking fabulous—not only by following the DASH Diet Younger You plan, but also by exercising in a specific way; managing your stress; and improving the quality of your sleep. All of these actions will lengthen your telomeres. Let's take a look at how.

Turn the Clock Back Ten Years:
The Anti-Aging Effect of Exercise

It's old news that exercise cuts your risk of obesity, heart disease, cancer, and other diseases, potentially extending your life. But exactly how? Answer: those cellular markers of aging, telomeres.

Cardio Exercise

Several years ago, researchers at King's College London measured what effect cardio exercise—the kind that gets your heart pumping—might have on telomere length. The team accessed a British health registry of 2,401 adult twins who had filled out detailed medical questionnaires. The twins had also donated blood, which the scientists could use to determine the length of their telomeres.

That length was directly related to the twins' activity levels. Those who exercised moderately—about 100 minutes a week of activity such as tennis, swimming, or running—had telomeres that were the length of people five or six years younger. Those who did the most exercise—doing about three hours a week of moderate to vigorous activity—had even longer telomeres. Clearly, as the amount of exercise increased, the telomere length increased. This study was published in the *Archives of Internal Medicine* in 2008.

You can take advantage of this scientific knowledge very easily. Start walking three to five times a week, at least thirty minutes each time. Gradually increase your intensity—level of effort—by walking faster, climbing a hill, or turning your walk into a slow jog. Cardio activity will trim your waistline, thus reducing your risk for diabetes, high blood pressure, and heart disease. Cardio boosts your circulation, too—a positive side effect that is very nourishing for your skin. Healthy circulation removes waste and toxins and brings healing oxygen and nutrients to your skin.

Cardio exercise will also strengthen your heart muscle, as well as other muscles in your body. Your heart can then pump blood more easily, and your blood pressure will go down. This type of exercise is a great stress reliever, too. It gives you something to focus on other than your problems. Exercise simply makes you feel better, whether it is a brisk thirty-minute walk or bicycle ride through the park, a hike in the woods, an hour of tennis, or a workout session in which you use all your muscles. There are a deep calm, a sense of accomplishment, and a mood-lifting effect after exercise that make you feel better all day.

Thus, with a simple cardio program, you'll start to look younger nearly right away.

Strength Training

Strength training—the application of muscle power against resistance—has long been known to break the age barrier. It prevents age-related declines in vulnerable hot spots: your muscles, bones, and metabolism. The stronger your muscles, bones, and metabolism are, the less likely age can prey on them and you. Now we're learning that, like cardio workouts, strength training can also lengthen those ever-so-important telomeres.

In 2008, Swedish researchers compared a group of power lifters, who had strength-trained for more than eight years, with a group of healthy, active subjects who had no history of strength training. Muscle biopsies were taken in order to study telomere length. The researchers found that telomeres were longer in the power lifters. Conclusion: Strength training does help lengthen telomeres. This study was published in *Medicine & Science in Sports & Exercise*.

A stronger body is simply a younger body. In one study, researchers from Tufts Center on Aging had people in their eighties and nineties working out on strength machines and lifting weights. In just eight weeks, these subjects shocked the researchers by throwing away their canes and walkers and moving with the posture and vigor of healthy people thirty years their juniors! The research, which was published in 1990 in the *Journal of the American Medical Association*, was so astounding that it has continued to influence much research on healthy aging and has shattered our views about what we can expect from the super-elderly.

I first became interested in strength training after reading Miriam E. Nelson's work *Strong Women Stay Young*. The premise of this book was to use strength training along with cardio to create younger bones. (And Dr. Nelson was part of that breakthrough Tufts research team!) Strength exercises, which include weight training and weight-bearing cardio exercises, are the best for rejuvenating our bones and muscles. I'm such a believer in strength training that I have free weights and ankle weights at home. I go to the gym weekly for high-intensity strength training. No, I don't have bulging muscles. But I'm firm and toned. I feel so much younger than most people I know, even those who are decades younger than me. And of course, the more muscle you have (and the more conditioned your muscles are), the faster your metabolism. This is a great way to keep your body leaner without resorting to starvation diets.

Flexibility

As strength can decline with age, so can flexibility—our ability to flex and extend our joints and the range of motion we need for basic movement. Rigidity and stiffness can start in our thirties, and they really start to speed up in later decades, unless we stretch regularly or do flexibility work such as Pilates, t'ai chi, or yoga as the years pass.

The question is: Does flexibility training affect telomeres in any way? Answer: Yes, if done in conjunction with a healthy diet that sharply reduces the amount of meat you eat—a diet like the DASH Diet Younger You plan. A study at the University of California, San Francisco—which I referred to earlier—looked into the effects of healthy living on telomeres in two groups of men who had early nonaggressive prostate cancer. Blood tests found that when they changed their diet, practiced yoga, and reduced their stress, the length of their telomeres increased.

I encourage you to take up flexibility activities to tune into the mental as well as the physical benefits of exercise. Yoga and Pilates do so much to improve strength, balance, and flexibility while reducing stress and anxiety. You can find workout programs on cable TV, in Internet videos, by buying or downloading a video, going to classes at a park district, community center, or a health club, or going to small studios with specialty programs. Today there are so many variations of yoga that you may not know where to start, but please do consider starting, perhaps with a beginners' class.

A similar, meditative form of exercise is t'ai chi. You can find videos to follow, or if you are lucky, find an outdoor class in a park.

Creating an Anti-Aging Exercise Program: Getting Started

Ideally, an anti-aging exercise program should focus on building cardio endurance, strength, and flexibility. Sounds like a lot, but it isn't. Nor does it have to be time-consuming. With a little bit of effort and commitment, you can develop all three. Take these steps to get there.

Step 1: Remove Barriers to Exercise

It's easy to come up with excuses for not exercising. Excuses are simply barriers in our own minds. Identify your own barriers, then create solutions to overcome them. Some examples:

Need new shoes? Buy them.

Don't like to exercise outside because you have allergies? Find a gym, school, or community facility with an indoor track or treadmills.

Can't find the time in your busy schedule? March in place in front of the TV at the end of the day. Walk around the building or the block when you get to work. Take a midmorning or mid-afternoon stroll around the office, which, by the way, will get rid of those late-afternoon blahs. If you spend a lot of time on the phone, stand up and pace around your office while you talk. If your kids are in group sports, walk around on the sidelines while they are having their games or practices.

Think exercise is boring? Get a dog and walk it. On weekends, ride your bike or go hiking. If you have access to a pool, swim and cool off at the same time. Go to local dances. I love going to places where I can do the Texas two-step and other country dances. Virtually every one of the dancers I've seen has a flat stomach. You can put on music at home and dance around in your living room, bedroom, or basement. Or join a dance class.

Have physical challenges? If you have trouble standing up for any length of time because of arthritis or other physical roadblocks, go to a gym or fitness center with a heated pool and do the water aerobics or just walk back and forth across the pool. Chair exercises and dancing in your chair are other ways to get moving if you have pain when standing. Watch an exercise video and do as much as you can. You can lose weight, get healthy, and feel younger by doing simple, fun movements while seated.

Need accountability? Join a class, work out with a friend, or hire a personal trainer. Doing so gives you an "appointment" with exercise. You're less likely to break that appointment than if you were just trying to squeeze in exercise when you could. If you're exercising on your own, set a schedule and make yourself a priority.

Step 2: Decide on Your Activities

Make exercise fun! It doesn't have to be drudgery. Simply find activities you enjoy in each of the three anti-aging categories. For cardio, it might be walking, swimming, dancing, or some of the activities I described in Step 1. For strength training, it might be working out with weights or attending a strength-training class that features music. For flexibility, it might be yoga, Pilates, a stretching class, or t'ai chi. If you enjoy something, you're more likely to stick to it.

I DASHed Aging!

I had never exercised much in the past. Then I started the DASH Diet Younger You plan. It definitely fueled my body for exercise. Now I work out thirty minutes a day, five days a week. I was terribly overweight, and don't even want to admit how much I weighed. After only six weeks of being on the plan, I lost twenty-seven pounds. This is the first plan on which I've been able to lose weight—and exercise.

—Karen F.

Step 3: Plan Your Week

As you get started, you might plan to:

- Walk (or do other cardio exercise) two or three times a week, for thirty minutes each time. After you get past twenty minutes, you are primarily burning fat. I think of this as the golden time, because it really changes your shape.
- Strength-train once or twice a week, for about thirty minutes each time.
- Do flexibility exercises twice a week, for thirty to sixty minutes each time.

To save time, you might do cardio and strength training in the same workout session.

Here's an example of one way to set up your weekly exercise schedule, but don't feel obligated to follow this particular plan; please make your own.

Anti-Aging Workout Schedule

Sunday	Monday	Tuesday	Wednesday	Thursday	Friday	Saturday
Rest	Strength training, followed by cardio	Rest	Flexibility, followed by cardio	Strength training, followed by cardio	Cardio	Flexibility, followed by cardio

Step 4: Challenge Yourself

To keep making gains in your endurance, strength, and flexibility, you can try several strategies. You might increase your *frequency*, the number of times you exercise each week; your *intensity*, how hard you push yourself while exercising; and your *time*, the total amount of time you spend exercising in one session. You can change up any of these three components to achieve better health and greater longevity.

Some examples: For frequency, you might add another day or two of exercise to your weekly schedule; for intensity, you could increase the speed of your walking or the poundage on your weights when strength training; and for time, you could add five or ten minutes to your workouts. Any one of these changes will yield positive benefits, as well as introduce new challenges and motivators into your workout.

Step 5: Focus on How Exercise Makes You Feel

Connect your mind and body by tuning into the natural high you get from exercising. As you work out, your body releases feel-good chemicals called endorphins, which are more powerful than morphine. Feel these coursing through your body, creating a

I DASHed Aging!

I recently competed in a triathlon, something I thought I'd never, ever be able to do. After all, I'm forty-three years old and weighed 233 pounds. The DASH Diet Younger You plan made it possible for me to train and compete for this sport. I dropped my weight down to a healthy, fit 139 pounds. The plan also eliminated my high blood pressure, and I no longer need meds. I've never followed a better plan in my life. It has been a lifesaver.

—Christy A.

natural high. Notice your breath and feel it going in and out. Assess how each muscle group is working during your activity. Remind yourself how healthy and strong you are. Be thankful that these body parts work so well. Being grateful has a way of providing motivation.

And if you find exercise to be boring, explore different ways to mix it up and make it interesting for you. I love music, and I forget that I'm exercising if I have my headphones pumping out my favorites. Some people like to read, listen to audiobooks, or watch television while exercising. Find different parks or different routes for running, walking, or biking. Combining things you already like to do with exercise makes it a pleasure to be more active.

I've always encouraged people to move more, not only for weight loss, but also to make their bodies feel younger. Having a fitter body improves your posture, making you look younger. Your skin will start to glow. You'll develop youthful curves and tone. You'll feel stronger, and everything you do in your daily life will feel easier. Chalk it up to your newfound youthful vigor.

Ommmm!

Stress can speed up the development of outward signs of aging, such as gray hair and wrinkles—a process you see in U.S. presidents while they're in office. As early as two years into their terms, their faces and their whiter hair show the effects of the stress from dealing with wars, natural disasters, economic calamities, and more.

There are internal signs of aging, too. Stress increases blood pressure and abnormal cholesterol levels, known contributors to aging. Also, scientists have found proof that people under high stress and pressure have shorter telomeres. In one study, volunteers who scored very high on an anxiety scale had telomere lengths similar to nonanxious women who were six years older, according to a report published July 11, 2012, in *PLOS ONE*. The take-home message here: Relieve stress and anxiety, and you could turn the aging clock back six years!

But is accelerated aging because of stress inevitable?

Not necessarily, if you take some steps to relieve it. Exercise is one of the best ways to manage stress, and that's important for fighting the aging process. Another excellent stress remedy is meditation. It even lengthens telomeres, according to a 2013 study published in *Brain, Behavior, and Immunity*. Scientists compared telomere length in a group of individuals experienced in Loving-Kindness Meditation (LKM), a practice derived from Buddhism, with a control group who had done no meditation. The LKM practitioners had longer telomeres than the controls.

What exactly is going on at the cellular level? Meditation increases levels of the enzyme telomerase, which protects telomeres from shortening. This finding certainly changed my view of meditation as simply a state of relaxation. It's an age eraser!

I've long been a fan of meditation. When I was much younger, I suffered from multiple types of headaches, every day. I had depression headaches (stiff, painful neck), tension headaches (headband squeezing), cluster headaches (four to five each day), and migraine with auras (visual disturbances). I went to a headache clinic and was put on medication. Although the drugs got things under control relatively fast, I still felt a slight "background" headache, and my heart rate began to skyrocket. I wanted to get off the medication.

The clinic taught me biofeedback and meditation. I learned to make the surface temperature of my fingers rise by imagining increased blood flow to my fingers and away from my brain. It was a powerful tool that eliminated the migraines.

I learned to meditate for fifteen to twenty minutes twice a day. At the clinic, electrodes were attached to my scalp to measure whether I was producing the right type of brain waves while meditating. I got so that I could easily slip into a deep meditative state, which increased my creativity and eliminated the tension, depression, and cluster headaches. To this day, if I start to get a headache (which happens maybe once a year), I can reverse it with meditation.

How can you do the same? Let me share some techniques.

First, find a quiet place, free from distractions, and sit or recline comfortably.

Next, imagine warm waves of water washing over you, starting with your head and moving downward, removing tension and stress. Visualize the waves moving across your shoulders and down your arms, washing the stress out through your fingertips. Then see the waves going down your waist and to your legs, where they empty the stress out through the bottoms of your feet.

Breathe more deeply, letting your chest rise and fall in an even rhythm. Feel the current of your breaths, long and sturdy, easing in and easing out.

Feel the sensation of sinking into your chair or your bed, with all your cares being washed away. Take at least twenty minutes to go through this meditation.

Another option is to visualize yourself on a warm beach in

the tropics, with gentle breezes wafting over you and warm waves lapping over your feet. Imagine that all your stress is being swept away and you are floating on the sand.

Prayer, especially ritual prayer, produces the same meditative response. Anything you enjoy and love can be a meditation, be it gardening, listening to music, or painting. Make a regular habit of meditating. It will go a long way to protect you from stress and even help you live longer.

Good Night

You know you need a good night's sleep, but did you know that it can help you live longer? That's right. In 2014, the medical journal *SLEEP* reported on a study of 154 adults, forty-five to seventy-seven years old. The study found that participants who regularly slept seven or more hours a night had longer telomeres than people who slept less. Just think: You can refashion your fate at the level of your DNA by getting a good night's sleep!

A good night's sleep is vital for your overall health, anyway. Another study, by researchers at the University of Chicago, published in *Sleep Medicine Review* in 2007, showed that healthy young men could develop symptoms of type 2 diabetes in just three nights of interrupted sleep. Apparently, sleep deprivation can increase inflammatory chemicals (cytokines) and cause a low-grade inflammation, which we know is associated with the onset of insulin resistance and diabetes. There are several possible reasons for this, according to the study. Sleep disturbances may worsen metabolic syndrome, a diabetes-like condition, as well as increasing cortisol (the stress hormone), blood pressure, and cholesterol. Sleep is also apparently involved in regulating several additional hormones, including thyroid hormone and growth hormone. When sleep is restricted, the nervous system responds by increasing another stress hormone, epinephrine, which may hinder sugar metabolism. Whatever the underlying factors, you want to avoid conditions that increase your risk of diabetes. It's a disease of aging that can cut short your life, and definitely your quality of life, if uncontrolled.

The amount and quality of your slumber is also linked to mental deterioration and Alzheimer's disease, according to a mound of studies. One study discovered that people with sleep apnea—a potentially serious disorder in which breathing repeatedly stops and starts during sleep—were more than twice as likely to develop cognitive problems or dementia as problem-free sleepers.

On a less serious note but a vainer one, a lack of sleep can be especially devastating to your skin. The next morning, after you have an especially short sleep time, check your skin in the mirror. It will be more wrinkled, it may look reddish, and the pores will be more pronounced. You need good-quality sleep to remove toxins and refresh your skin.

Here are my suggestions for improving the quality and duration of your sleep:

- Shut down electronic devices. About thirty minutes before bedtime, put away your computer and phone and shut off the TV. Apparently, the light emanating from these devices wreaks havoc with our natural rhythms and confuses the mind into thinking it has to keep running, even though you would like it to shut down. Instead, try reading a book, sharing loving moments with your partner, meditating, or doing some stretching exercises, all of which are great ways to promote sound sleep.
- Watch your alcohol intake. Too much alcohol interferes with sleep patterns. Although you may fall asleep more quickly, your sleep quality will be poor, and you'll probably wake up a few times during the night. And the next morning, you will have that telltale poor skin appearance, with more

pronounced wrinkles and pores. The appearance problem is twofold: Alcohol dehydrates your skin and dilates surface blood vessels. So for your skin, your health, and your sleep, try to keep your alcohol consumption to no more than one or two drinks a night.

- Stick to a regular sleep schedule. If you're going to bed at different times every night, you're throwing off your body's natural rhythm. Be consistent in when you wake up and go to bed. If you do, you'll start feeling sleepy around the same time every night and wake up about the same time every morning because your body's biological clock won't be disrupted.

- Watch evening snacks. It's not a good idea to eat anything or chug liquids at least two hours before it's time for you to lie down. Going to bed on a full stomach makes digestion difficult and can aggravate heartburn, making it hard, and sometimes impossible, for your body to relax. Some doctors believe late-night eating can lead to weight gain. Your body is less sensitive to insulin at night and thus is more likely to store excess sugar in the fat cells around your waist, especially if you eat high-carb meals late at night.

- Take a warm bath one to two hours before bedtime. A warm bath soothes your body's muscles and makes it easier to relax. Conversely, a cooling evening shower on those hot summer days may help make it easier to fall asleep at bedtime.

- Make your sleeping environment comfortable. If you wear pajamas, wear comfy ones. Also, keep your room as cool as you can tolerate; your body goes to sleep better and has a deeper sleep in a colder temperature.

It's exciting to know that we have so much control over our own aging process—through what we eat, how we exercise, the way we manage stress, and how well we sleep. Lifestyle certainly equals longevity.

CHAPTER 10

Stop the Diseases of Aging

The killer illnesses we read about or that have affected us personally—heart disease, many cancers, diabetes, dementia, and others—are really diseases of aging. That's because the culprit behind virtually all of these diseases is cellular damage, brought on by oxidation, inflammation, and glycation. Eventually, this cellular damage weakens cells, organs, and other parts of our bodies, and we become older and sick.

As I hope you know by now, you can turn back this lethal process—with the DASH Diet Younger You plan. As previously mentioned, the DASH approach has been ranked as the Best Diet, the Healthiest Diet, and the Best Diet for multiple years by a panel of expert medical professionals assembled by *U.S. News & World Report*. Why is the DASH diet such a standout? Because it's the only diet ever to be researched so thoroughly and to consistently prove its merits over time.

Those merits are astounding. The DASH diet was developed primarily to reverse hypertension, and it was hoped that it would also lower cholesterol—and that it does. The diet has been proven to significantly reduce the risk of stroke, heart attack, type 2 diabetes, and some types of cancer—all diseases of aging.

Who wouldn't want to adopt this kind of eating plan?

Maybe you have a family history of some of these diseases and you're afraid that your golden years might be doomed, that there's not much you can do about it. Think again! Sure, you may have genes that make it more likely that you'll develop a disease of aging, but don't worry, because diet can improve your true destiny. Diet, along with lifestyle, can actually change how genes act, and turn off the bad ones. You stay younger and healthier from the inside out. Your future is truly in your hands.

Advice for preventing the diseases of aging often hinges on sole nutrients or single foods—for example: Eat blueberries…or cherries…or beans…or salmon…ad infinitum. It is more important to fit these foods into the DASH pattern of eating. By pattern, I mean a full variety of foods with which you plan your meals. It's not about eating blueberries all day long, to the exclusion of other fruits, because you want to prevent cancer or dementia; it's about eating blueberries maybe several times a week within the context of the DASH Diet Younger You plan.

With this in mind, let's look more closely at the diseases of aging and the foods and strategies you will want to emphasize within the healing pattern of DASH for each disease. I call these foods and strategies the age reversers.

Coronary Artery Disease

Coronary artery disease occurs when "plaque" begins to amass inside the arteries that encircle the heart. These arteries are as small as the inside of a piece of dry macaroni. Plaque narrows the arteries, and a blood clot can form or a piece of plaque can break off at the site of the narrowing, setting off a heart attack.

To prevent coronary artery disease and heart attacks, you've got to decrease LDL cholesterol (low-density lipoprotein cholesterol, or "bad" cholesterol) and triglycerides. The LDL also contains a fraction known as VLDL (very-low-density lipoprotein cholesterol), which is even more likely to clog up your arteries. And, even worse, when LDL gets oxidized, always a major aging process, it is most likely to create plaque.

Unfortunately, age can unbalance your coronary health, and your body can gradually shift into a chronically inflamed state called inflamm-aging, and into chronic oxidative stress, called oxid-aging. Both of these issues are addressed by the DASH Diet Younger You plan, since it is rich in anti-inflammatory foods and antioxidants to help protect your heart. In fact, research has shown that people following the DASH diet have an approximately 30 percent reduction in their ten-year risk of having a heart attack.

Triglycerides (blood fats) will plug up your blood vessels, too. In addition, high levels indicate that you're at increased risk for developing type 2 diabetes. Occasionally, someone will not be diagnosed with high triglycerides until the level is quite high, up toward 1,000 mg/dL. The blood will actually appear milky from the high level of these fats in the blood. Another complication: When triglycerides are high, blood tests can't read LDL numbers.

Classifications of Blood Lipid Levels

New guidelines for cholesterol and triglycerides (lipids) are still up in the air, with a lot of controversy surrounding their development and new recommendations. Here I present the cholesterol guidelines that have been in effect for some time, since they will probably be the ones used by your physician.

(continued)

Total Cholesterol

Desirable: <200
Borderline high: 200–239
High: 240+

LDL Cholesterol

Desirable with CVD (Cardiovascular disease): <70
Optimal: <100
Near or above optimal: 100–129
Borderline high: 130–159
High: 160–189
Very high: 190+

HDL Cholesterol

Low: <40
High (desirable): 60+

Triglycerides (Triacylglycerols)

Normal: <150
Borderline high: 150–199
High: 200–499
Very high: 500+

When Good Cholesterol Goes Bad

A high number is good when you're talking about your HDL (high-density lipoprotein). You can make it easy to remember which one is the good cholesterol by remembering "H" for "healthy" or for "high." And you can remember "L" for "low," since you want the bad cholesterol, LDL, to be low. Like all forms of cholesterol, HDL is wrapped in protein packages that help move it through the bloodstream. HDL is beneficial, whereas LDL can be deadly. In fact, HDL sweeps around your arteries like a vacuum, cleaning up cholesterol from plaque.

I have seen so many patients who thought they were following their doctors' advice for healthy eating but found that their HDL had dropped like a rock. They were so disappointed, because they thought they were doing everything right.

On analyzing their diets, we found out that they were overeating foods high in added sugar and refined starch. A diet like this will produce more triglycerides in many people. The packaging for the triglycerides (called chylomicrons) soaks up some of the cholesterol from the HDL, which shrinks them, thus reducing their weight and making the HDL reading go down. The more triglycerides, the lower HDL is likely to be.

This is why a diet high in refined starchy or added-sugar foods causes your HDL to go down. Unfortunately, this is the direct result of outdated diet advice that encouraged people to cut way back on fat and increase their intake of grains. Not only does this eating pattern make you susceptible to heart disease, it also increases your chances of developing nonalcoholic fatty liver disease (which is approaching epidemic rates, having doubled in prevalence over the past fifteen years). This disease is an accumulation of fat within your liver and can progress either to cirrhosis or to liver cancer.

Age Reversers for Coronary Heart Disease

- Make sure to eat nuts and heart-healthy fats (especially extra virgin olive oil and fatty cold-water fish like salmon and tuna). These are all part of the DASH Diet Younger You plan. These foods help lower bad cholesterol and triglycerides while boosting HDL.

- Avoid saturated fats and trans fats; both are artery cloggers. To do so, eat only lean meats and avoid processed foods (which can be high in trans fats and saturated fats). Fortunately, all the fiber you'll be eating will help soak up bad fats and whisk them out of your body.
- Limit your consumption of red meats to two or three times or less a week. Choose lean cuts. Trim away visible fat after cooking. Prepare the meat without adding fat.
- Avoid processed or luncheon meats, sausages, and bacon. They are full of salt, which is aging for your heart.
- As an alternative to red meat, it's fine to choose poultry or fish. Other excellent sources of protein are beans and peas—lentils, kidney beans, chickpeas, and others.
- Don't skimp on dairy. The calcium in dairy foods binds to fats and reduces their absorption.
- Avoid starchy refined foods and those with added sugars, as they will increase your triglycerides. On the other hand, fish and other foods with omega-3s will reduce triglycerides.
- Eat from the rainbow. Colorful plant-based foods will reduce inflammation of the linings of your arteries. And those same fruits, veggies, and nuts are packed with antioxidants that reduce the oxidation of cholesterol, making it less likely to clog arteries.

Blood Pressure

Hypertension has been called the silent disease because it usually has no symptoms. One in every three adult Americans has hypertension or high blood pressure, and many don't even know it. And another 25 percent have prehypertension. Even if you have normal blood pressure at age fifty, you have a 90 percent chance of developing hypertension during your lifetime. If you're taking oral contraceptives, you are two to three times more likely to have high blood pressure. When your blood pressure is high over time, it makes you more prone to stroke, coronary artery disease, heart failure, and kidney disease.

And unfortunately, hypertension is not an equal-opportunity disease. Your geographic region and ethnicity can have a major impact on your risk for blood pressure. People in the southeastern United States have much higher rates, which leads to this region's designation as the Stroke Belt. African-Americans are more likely to die from heart disease, are more likely to have quality-of-life-compromising consequences of high blood pressure and heart disease, and to suffer from faster progression of these diseases. Currently, 44 percent of adult African-Americans have hypertension.

Understanding Your Blood Pressure Reading

Systolic blood pressure		Diastolic blood pressure	Classification
90–119	And	60–79	Desirable blood pressure
120–139	Or	80–89	Prehypertension
140–159	Or	90–99	Stage 1 hypertension
160 or higher	Or	100 or higher	Stage 2 hypertension

If you're at risk, take heart. The DASH Diet Younger You plan lowers blood pressure quickly—within just two weeks—as well as do the first-line blood pressure medications. And people with more advanced disease can see improved blood pressure control, too, because DASH can help them respond better to their medication.

This is extremely important, since only half of people with high blood pressure have it under control.

The DASH Diet Younger You plan is rich in magnesium, potassium, calcium, and fiber—all of which work synergistically to lower blood pressure. If you have high blood pressure, be sure to do the following after you go on the DASH Diet Younger You plan:

Age Reversers for High Blood Pressure

- Make sure your food choices are high in potassium. Examples include milk, bananas, potatoes, and oranges. Potassium helps flush out excess sodium. See Appendix C for a list of high potassium foods.
- Eat foods high in vitamins C and D. Both nutrients help relax blood vessels, allowing for better blood flow so the heart doesn't have to pump as hard. This strategy keeps your blood pressure under control. Foods rich in vitamin C include citrus fruits; those rich in vitamin D include dairy foods and some fish.
- Corral some calcium. More than two decades have come and gone since researchers first suggested that calcium in drinking water was related to lower blood pressure. And over the years, the calcium-hypertension link has grown stronger. In fact, in the original DASH research, the blood pressure reductions were not obtained just by consuming more fruits and vegetables; dairy was necessary to get the full blood pressure benefits. Adults need 1,000 milligrams of calcium a day for good health; after age fifty, up the amount to 1,200 milligrams a day. Food sources include dairy, sardines, kale, collards, mustard greens, and other dark-green leafy vegetables.

- Look to magnesium. This mineral has a positive effect on errant blood pressure, too. You can get adequate magnesium from many food sources, including dark-green leafy vegetables, nuts, beans, and whole grains.
- Drop some weight. One of the most powerful ways to lower blood pressure is to lose weight or stay at a healthy weight. When your weight goes down, so does your blood pressure. In addition to following the DASH diet, use exercise to shed pounds. It also keeps your blood vessels flexible—a must for blood pressure control.

I DASHed Aging!

Late last year, I rushed myself to the local Urgent Care for bronchitis. My blood pressure was 190/90. I was horrified and knew I needed to take charge of my health. I have two young children, and I want to be there for them as they grow up. I researched diets, knowing I needed something I could maintain for the rest of my life. Going back to my old habits was not an option for me.

I learned about DASH on the *U.S. News & World Report* and Mayo Clinic websites. I immediately purchased Marla Heller's books. At the time, I needed a primary physician (mine had moved), so I scheduled a new-patient appointment, but that took about six weeks. Nonetheless, I started DASH right away.

By the time I finally saw the doctor, I had lost about twenty-four pounds. My blood pressure was down to 140/86. Unfortunately, my blood work revealed that I had diabetes.

(continued)

Undeterred, I stuck with the plan. To date, I have lost forty pounds by following DASH and exercising about thirty minutes, five days a week. My blood pressure is normal—usually around 112/76 or lower—and my blood sugar is well controlled. I have more energy, no cravings, and I find the diet very easy to follow. A couple of weeks ago, I put my keys in my pocket and my size 22 pants literally fell to my ankles. I was very happy that didn't happen while I was out!

My husband is also on the plan, and he is losing weight, too. The key for me is to be prepared, bring healthy snacks with me when I am out for hours, and keep DASH-friendly ingredients in the house. I have about sixty more pounds to lose, and I have no doubt that I will achieve my goal.

—Amy W.

Stroke

Each year 800,000 Americans have a stroke. Often referred to as a brain attack, a stroke is a blockage or rupture in the arteries leading to the brain, in which the supply of blood, oxygen, and glucose to the brain is cut off.

The better controlled your blood pressure is, the lower your risk of stroke. In a large-scale study following more than 90,000 nurses for over twenty-five years, a DASH-style eating pattern was associated with a 17 percent lower risk of stroke compared with women following a less healthful eating pattern. This is an important finding, since one American woman in every five will have a stroke during her lifetime—a slightly higher risk than for men.

Strokes can be debilitating, and many people never fully recover. A stroke ages a person fast; it can lead to depression and hinder the ability to fully enjoy life.

If you might be at risk for stroke, you definitely want to follow the DASH Diet Younger You plan—and emphasize the following strategies as part of the plan.

Age Reversers to Prevent Stroke

- Color yourself protected. High-flavonoid foods slashed stroke risk dramatically, according to a report in the *Archives of Internal Medicine*, in 1996.
- Kick the nicotine habit. Smoking increases your odds of stroke by as much as 400 percent and is one of the top preventable risk factors.
- Get off the couch. Following a regular exercise program, such as brisk walking or even calisthenics, can reduce your risk of stroke by 63 percent, according to the American Academy of Neurology. (See Chapter 9 for advice on how to start an anti-aging exercise program.)

Metabolic Syndrome

Most people don't know what metabolic syndrome is, but huge numbers of Americans have it—about one out of every three adults.

Metabolic syndrome is a constellation of symptoms:

- Blood pressure that is higher than the optimal range
- High triglycerides
- Excess weight around the waist
- Higher-than-optimal blood sugar
- Lower-than-optimal HDL levels

To be diagnosed with metabolic syndrome, you need to have only three out of five of these symptoms (see the chart below).

Metabolic Syndrome Diagnosis (U.S.) with 3 or More of the Following

Triglycerides	Over 150
Waist circumference	Over 40 inches (102 cm) for men
	Over 35 inches (88 cm) for women
Low HDL	Less than 40 mg/dL for men
	Less than 50 mg/dL for women
Elevated blood pressure	Greater than 130 mm Hg SBP or 85 mm Hg DBP or on medication for blood pressure
Elevated fasting blood glucose	Greater than 110 mg/dL

Metabolic syndrome is a sure sign that you're aging before your time. It indicates that your body isn't metabolizing sugar and carbohydrates as well as when you were younger, and thus, you're at a higher risk of developing type 2 diabetes. Most of the symptoms I've listed above are signs of poor sugar metabolism—and an aging body.

The DASH Diet Younger You plan addresses all five symptoms of metabolic syndrome. Your blood pressure will be reduced. So will your triglycerides and blood sugar. Your HDL will improve. You'll get your weight under control, in part, as a result of getting your blood sugar numbers into a healthy range.

If you have metabolic syndrome or are headed in that direction, emphasize the following in the DASH Diet Younger You plan:

Age Reversers for Metabolic Syndrome

- Make sure to eat the required amounts of fruits and vegetables, nuts, seeds, legumes, and dairy. These foods address and correct all five symptoms of metabolic syndrome.
- For seeds, add pumpkin seeds to your plan. They're high in magnesium. A magnesium-rich diet may also help reduce the risk of metabolic syndrome.
- Get in the zinc sync. Zinc-rich foods have been shown to keep metabolic syndrome in check. Oysters, crabmeat, lean grass-fed beef, and dark chocolate are all good food sources of zinc.

Type 2 Diabetes

It's a sad but true statistic: Diabetes has skyrocketed to epidemic levels in this country. One out of every four Americans has prediabetes, and 16 percent have type 2 diabetes, and of those, only half even know it.

Diabetes is a serious disease of aging. It brings with it an increased risk of several other age-related diseases, such as heart attack, stroke, and premature death. What's more, chronically high blood sugar levels often damage the tiny blood vessels in the eyes, kidneys, and nerves. You can gradually lose your eyesight, kidney function, and sensation in your limbs. Poorly controlled diabetes has been shown to reduce life expectancy by ten to fifteen years.

Diabetes is a progressive disease. You can speed it up considerably with the wrong choices. Some examples: eating lots of low-fiber, high-starch, or high-added-sugar foods; consuming foods high in saturated fats and trans fats; not eating enough antioxidant and anti-inflammatory foods; and being inactive.

Optimal blood sugar level is about 75 to 80 if you have been fasting; however, it is considered normal as long as the fasting level is less than 100. Prediabetes is the range of 100 to 125, which is one of the hallmarks of metabolic syndrome. Full-blown diabetes can be diagnosed if your fasting blood sugar is 126 or higher on more than one occasion, and/or if your glucose is over 200 after two oral glucose tolerance tests (OGTTs). Physicians will also evaluate A1c (glycosylated hemoglobin—and yes, this is one of those measures of glyco-aging) as a way of measuring how well your blood sugar has been controlled over the most recent three-month period, and they can use this to diagnose diabetes. You may be considered to have prediabetes if you have an A1c of 5.7 to 6.4. If it is 6.5 or higher, you may be diagnosed with diabetes.

Finding out you have diabetes can be scary. But these days, doctors and dietitians are doling out a lot of good news about fighting it. Diabetes may not be curable, but it is manageable. And if you are concerned about getting the disease, it can be preventable. You can stop it before it gets started.

Following the DASH diet helps you both control the disease and prevent it. One chief reason is that you'll be cutting out refined starches, sugars, and low-fiber foods. As a result, you won't have as much glucose surging into your bloodstream. That way, it's much easier for your body to produce sufficient insulin to move the sugar out of the blood and into your muscles for energy. With normalized blood sugar, your liver won't be forced into making triglycerides in an attempt to help out, and your triglycerides will go back to normal. Nor will your liver stockpile fat, reversing fatty liver disease. Your belly will shrink because there's no excess sugar to soak up and deposit as fat around your middle. In effect, the DASH Diet Younger You plan stops the cascade of events that leads to diabetes, or hastens its progression.

Here are strategies to emphasize on the DASH Diet Younger You plan to prevent diabetes or tame it once it surfaces.

Age Reversers for Diabetes

- Don't skimp on fruits and vegetables. They prevent inflammation and oxidation from harming your tissues, organs, and blood vessels, all of which are in jeopardy with diabetes. These food groups helps heal your pancreas so it can continue to produce insulin for your entire life.

- Cut way back on any processed grains, such as in many cereals and breads. These starches can wear out the pancreas' ability to produce enough insulin, directly causing type 2 diabetes. Instead, emphasize high-fiber foods, including whole grains, nuts, beans, vegetables, and fruits. These high-fiber foods help your body metabolize sugar and insulin more efficiently.

- Mine for magnesium. This mineral can help protect against diabetes, and it is amply supplied in the DASH Diet Younger You plan. Some of the best food sources for magnesium are sunflower seeds, quinoa, spinach, almonds, brown rice, beans, and avocados.

- Get off bad fats. Reducing saturated fat and focusing on a plant-based diet like the DASH Diet might help you reduce your medication use, if you already have diabetes. In a study of 40,000 male health professionals who were followed over twenty years, it was found that the subjects had a 46 percent lower risk of developing diabetes by following the DASH diet.

- Get moving. Exercise is a major weapon against diabetes. It helps cells use insulin more efficiently and is critical to blood sugar control.

(Note: If you have diabetes, consult your physician and/or dietitian before you make major changes in your diet or modify your medications. This is especially important if you are on insulin.)

I DASHed Aging!

I got the shock of my life one day when my doctor called to tell me that my blood sugar test showed a severe elevation: 149. He wanted me to come in and have a fasting glucose test to check for diabetes. I agreed to the test, saying I would get it done within two months. I thought the first test was a mistake or a fluke.

Around the same time, my husband and I decided to lose weight to make ourselves healthier. I had read about the DASH plan online, so I purchased the book to get started.

I decided to test my blood sugar at home just prior to starting the diet. It was a staggering 164. This was a real wake-up call. I was terrified. I did not want to be sick with a scary disease like diabetes.

Right away, my husband and I started "DASHing." We went grocery shopping and cut out all of our typical junk. We loaded up on fresh vegetables and started eating healthy that same day. Within the first two weeks I joined the online support community for DASH.

Not only did I see my blood sugar slowly come down, I also saw pounds melt off. I felt so much better! I had a headache in that first week and found out that my body was going through withdrawal and losing its addiction to salt and sugar.

My goal was to lose 10 percent of my body weight and see if my blood sugar would stabilize. If so, I'd go to the doctor and get tested for diabetes. Well, only five weeks after starting DASH, I retested my blood sugar, and it was a very respectable 92. What a miracle!

I've changed not only the way I look at food but also the way I look at my health. We can be in control. DASH is for life.

> As for my husband, his blood pressure is lower.
> Consequently, he needs his blood pressure medication
> reevaluated. Plus, he has lost thirty pounds.
>
> I've lost twenty-one pounds to date. My goal is to continue
> to lose weight until I get to my final goal. I have other
> goals, however. I do not want my son and daughter to have
> to remember me as fat. I want to live a long time, enjoy my
> grandchildren, and play with them without getting out of
> breath. I want to live!
>
> —Jessie L.

Dementia

Your brain changes with age. Over the years, brain weight and volume decrease. In fact, between age twenty and age ninety, the brain loses 5 to 10 percent of its weight.

But getting older isn't the only reason your brain becomes smaller. Your lifestyle matters, too. Researchers collected data on more than 1,300 middle-aged people participating in the Framingham Offspring Cohort Study and discovered that chronic health conditions, such as diabetes, and bad habits, such as smoking, can accelerate brain shrinkage.

Bad habits can also trigger other changes. For instance, poor diet and lack of exercise can clog arteries, even those leading to the brain. When these arteries are obstructed, the brain doesn't get a normal supply of blood, oxygen, or nutrients. It's starved, in other words, and that can increase your risk for dementia. In addition, the aging brain has a hard time defending itself against the inflammation and free radical damage inflicted by harmful habits.

If these processes are allowed to progress unchecked, dementia can set in. Dementia is the gradual loss of memory, thinking, and problem-solving skills, and a general decline in brainpower. Alzheimer's disease is a form of dementia.

Fortunately, research shows you can dodge dementia, or at least lower your risk, by following DASH. One of the main ways DASH helps preserve brainpower is by reducing the oxidative stress that causes premature aging of the brain.

Remember, oxidation is like rusting. When metal rusts, it weakens and flakes; it starts to degenerate or decay, until it no longer holds up. Eventually, the metal "fatigues" and "fails." This same process happens in our brains! DASH is loaded with antioxidants that help prevent this process. It is well known that powerful antioxidant foods, such as the berries found in the DASH diet, help slow cognitive decline.

If you have diabetes, you're more likely to develop dementia. That's because of damage to arteries and to the small blood vessels that bring nourishment and oxygen to your brain, and because of interference with glucose metabolism, since glucose is the main fuel for your brain. By keeping blood sugar under control with DASH and exercise, you prevent diabetes, and in doing so, prevent dementia.

High blood pressure is known to be particularly damaging to the brain. Besides being the major factor in causing strokes, clogged arteries reduce the flow of oxygen to the brain. In 2013, researchers from Rush University in Chicago reported at the Alzheimer's Association International Conference that they had seen an inverse relationship (lower risk) between how closely people followed a DASH diet eating pattern and their risk of developing dementia. A similar 2013 study at Utah State University also saw a strong association with improved preservation of brainpower over eleven years in people who were following a DASH eating pattern.

Here's a look at what else you can do to keep your brain young, alert, and laser-sharp for life.

Age Reversers for Dementia

- Add sources of omega-3 fatty acids, such as salmon, tuna, and walnuts, to your diet. These foods can help preserve brain volume and slow the shrinkage of the brain, thus keeping your brain much younger.
- Use the D defense. People who are deficient in vitamin D are 42 percent more likely to have cognitive impairment, and the chance is almost 400 percent higher if the deficiency is severe. Since most Americans are deficient in vitamin D, especially during the winter months, the milk and yogurt in the DASH diet can be a huge benefit.
- Shed pounds. Weight loss or being at a healthy weight helps. A study of bariatric surgery patients found that their weight loss was associated with improved memory.
- Stay plant-focused. The fruits and vegetables on the DASH diet are full of antioxidants and anti-inflammatories to keep your brain younger.
- Say yes to blueberries. Despite their small size, blueberries are a powerful defense against oxidative stress, which ages your body and your brain. The red pigments, or anthocyanins, in blueberries and other berries are nutritional heroes, according to a study released by Tufts University. Blueberries also help your brain manufacture dopamine as you age. Dopamine is a naturally occurring brain chemical that is crucial for memory, muscular coordination, and general well-being.
- Work out. Get moving with some kind of physical activity for at least thirty minutes daily. Aim for at least five days each week and you will be doing your best to keep a young brain. Physical activity is the best vaccine against dementia.

Cancer

Cancer is primarily a disease of aging, with the majority of cancer cases being diagnosed in people over fifty. The reasons, however, are unclear, since cancer is such a complicated disease.

It's clearer to scientists that the DASH diet lowers the risk of developing colorectal cancer and ER− (estrogen-receptor-negative) breast cancer. Of course, a diet rich in fruits and vegetables, like the DASH diet, is associated with lower risk of all types of cancers, thanks to the anticancer, DNA-protective action of flavonoids and antioxidants. Some of these plant components even hasten the death of cancer cells.

As you've probably realized, you'll lose weight on the DASH Diet Younger You plan. Not only will this help you look good and feel better about yourself, but you'll also lower your odds of cancer. That's because obesity is associated with increased risk for several types of cancer, including ovarian and breast cancers.

Is Your Weight in a Healthy Range?

Body Mass Index (BMI) is a good way to find out. You can determine your BMI by going to dashdiet.org/healthy_weight.asp or checking the chart in Appendix B. The information below will show you where you stand.

BMI	Classification
Less than 19	Underweight
19–24.9	Desirable weight
25–29.9	Overweight
30 and higher	Obese

You'll be eating little refined sugar on this plan—an action that further protects you against cancer. Cancer cells love to feed on sugar. Cutting off their sugar supply is an effective cancer-fighting strategy.

And by choosing unprocessed and minimally processed foods, without added hormones, pesticides, or packaging additives, you can minimize cancer-promoting toxins that enter your system.

Let's get down to some specifics in terms of preventing this dreaded disease of aging.

Age Reversers for Cancer

- Enjoy broccoli. This veggie contains two powerful anticancer phytochemicals, sulforaphane and indole-3-carbinol. Sulforaphane works in two ways. First, it destroys any carcinogens that you've eaten, and second, it manufactures enzymes that clean up any carcinogens left over from that reaction. Indole-3-carbinol helps your body metabolize excess estrogen, which can cause breast cancer. And the other veggies in this food group have similar cancer-fighting properties. They include cauliflower, cabbage, radishes, mustard greens, and Brussels sprouts.

- Go for some onions. They may make your breath stink, but onions are a standout in the anticancer arena. Plenty of research links onions to a reduced risk of certain cancers, namely breast, esophagus, and stomach cancers. Researchers suspect that the flavonoid quercetin, along with the organosulfur compounds (associated with the onion smell), are largely responsible for the cancer-fighting ability of onions.

- Fall in love with tomatoes. Dozens of large-scale studies have reported that eating a lot of tomatoes is highly protective against all sorts of cancer, particularly prostate, lung, and stomach cancer. Lycopene, a carotenoid found in tomatoes, seems to be the main reason for the anticancer benefit.

225

- Stay active. Exercise has proven in research to be a great ally in the fight against cancer, particularly breast cancer. Exercise, of course, burns body fat. Researchers have known for some time that fatter women make more estrogen, and more potent forms of estrogen that have been related to increased cancers of the reproductive system. It's likely that lean women make less estrogen, and less potent estrogen. Staying lean through exercise confers a definite protective benefit.

You Can Do It

Blood pressure down! Blood sugar down! Cholesterol down! Triglycerides down! And of course, waist size down! And then you ARE younger, from the inside out.

The simple truth is that you can stay young, or become young again. To sum up everything I've said in this book, I'll say this to you: Use the right foods to rejuvenate yourself. Move your body to regenerate it. Tap into the natural process of self-renewal with sleep and stress management. Do the things that keep you young.

Make a start, and I'll bet you'll be a younger you very soon.

U.S. to Metric Conversions

U.S. to Metric Conversions, Height

Inches	Centimeters	Inches	Centimeters	Inches	Centimeters
58	147	67	170	76	193
59	150	68	173	77	196
60	152	69	175	78	198
61	155	70	178	79	201
62	157	71	180	80	203
63	160	72	183	81	206
64	163	73	185	82	208
65	165	74	188		
66	168	75	191		

U.S. to Metric Conversions, Weight

Pounds	Kilograms
½ (8 ounces)	0.23
1 (16 ounces)	0.45
1½	0.68
2	0.91
2½	1.13
3	1.36

U.S., Imperial, and Metric Conversions, Weight

Pounds	Stones	Kilograms	Pounds	Stones	Kilograms
95	6.8	43.1	195	13.9	88.5
100	7.1	45.4	200	14.3	90.7
105	7.5	47.6	205	14.6	93.0
110	7.9	49.9	210	15.0	95.3
115	8.2	52.2	215	15.4	97.5
120	8.6	54.4	220	15.7	99.8
125	8.9	56.7	225	16.1	102.1
130	9.3	59.0	230	16.4	104.3
135	9.6	61.2	235	16.8	106.6
140	10.0	63.5	240	17.1	108.9
145	10.4	65.8	245	17.5	111.1
150	10.7	68.0	250	17.9	113.4
155	11.1	70.3	255	18.2	115.7
160	11.4	72.6	260	18.6	117.9
165	11.8	74.8	265	18.9	120.2
170	12.1	77.1	270	19.3	122.5
175	12.5	79.4	275	19.6	124.7
180	12.9	81.6	280	20.0	127.0
185	13.2	83.9	285	20.4	129.3
190	13.6	86.2	290	20.7	131.5

Pounds	Stones	Kilograms	Pounds	Stones	Kilograms
295	21.1	133.8	325	23.2	147.4
300	21.4	136.1	330	23.6	149.7
305	21.8	138.3	335	23.9	152.0
310	22.1	140.6	340	24.3	154.2
315	22.5	142.9	345	24.6	156.5
320	22.9	145.1	350	25.0	158.8

U.S. to Metric Conversions, Temperature

Degrees Fahrenheit	Degrees Celsius
300	149
325	163
350	177
375	191
400	204
425	218
450	232
475	246

U.S. to Metric Conversions, Volume
(Dry and Liquid)

Teaspoons	Milliliters
¼	1
½	2
1	5
3 (1 tablespoon)	15
6 (2 tablespoons)	30

U.S. to Metric Conversions, Volume (Liquid)

Fluid Ounces	Milliliters
1	30
2	60
3	90
4	120
5	150
6	180
7	210
8	240

The following information is provided as a point of reference:

U.S. Conversions, Volume

3 teaspoons = 1 tablespoon

2 tablespoons = 1 fluid ounce

8 fluid ounces = 1 cup

2 cups = 1 pint

2 pints = 1 quart

Imperial Conversions, Volume

10 fluid ounces = 1 cup

20 fluid ounces = 1 pint

40 fluid ounces = 1 quart

Note: Since this book does not contain any baking recipes (such as pastries, breads, cakes), precision is not important with the quantities. Typically in U.S. recipes, volumes, rather than weights, are used for most ingredients.

APPENDIX B

BMI (Body Mass Index)

Height (inches)	18	19	20	21	22	23	24	25	26	27	28	29	30	31	32	33	34	35	36	37	38	39	40
58	86	91	96	100	105	110	115	120	124	129	134	139	144	148	153	158	163	167	172	177	182	187	191
59	89	94	99	104	109	114	119	124	129	134	139	144	149	153	158	163	168	173	178	183	188	193	198
60	92	97	102	108	113	118	123	128	133	138	143	148	154	159	164	169	174	179	184	189	195	200	205
61	95	101	106	111	116	122	127	132	138	143	148	153	159	164	169	175	180	185	191	196	201	206	212
62	98	104	109	115	120	126	131	137	142	148	153	159	164	169	175	180	186	191	197	202	208	213	219
63	102	107	113	119	124	130	135	141	147	152	158	164	169	175	181	186	192	198	203	209	215	220	226
64	105	111	117	122	128	134	140	146	151	157	163	169	175	181	186	192	198	204	210	216	221	227	233
65	108	114	120	126	132	138	144	150	156	162	168	174	180	186	192	198	204	210	216	222	228	234	240
66	112	118	124	130	136	142	149	155	161	167	173	180	186	192	198	204	211	217	223	229	235	242	248
67	115	121	128	134	140	147	153	160	166	172	178	185	192	198	204	211	217	223	230	236	243	249	255
68	118	125	132	138	145	151	158	164	171	178	184	191	197	204	210	217	224	230	237	243	250	256	263
69	122	129	135	142	149	156	163	169	176	183	190	196	203	210	217	223	230	237	244	251	257	264	271
70	125	132	139	146	153	160	167	174	181	188	195	202	209	216	223	230	237	244	251	258	265	272	279
71	129	136	143	151	158	165	172	179	186	194	201	208	215	222	229	237	244	251	258	265	272	280	287
72	133	140	147	155	162	170	177	184	192	199	206	214	221	229	236	243	251	258	265	273	280	288	295
73	136	144	152	159	167	174	182	189	197	205	212	220	227	235	243	250	258	265	273	280	288	296	303
74	140	148	156	164	171	179	187	195	203	210	218	226	234	241	249	257	265	273	280	288	296	304	312
75	144	152	160	168	176	184	192	200	208	216	224	232	240	248	256	264	272	280	288	296	304	312	320
76	148	156	164	173	181	189	197	205	214	222	230	238	246	255	263	271	279	288	296	304	312	320	329
77	152	160	169	177	186	194	202	211	219	228	236	245	253	261	270	278	287	295	304	312	320	329	337
78	156	164	173	182	190	199	208	216	225	234	242	251	260	268	277	286	294	303	312	320	329	337	346
79	160	169	178	186	195	204	213	222	231	240	249	257	266	275	284	293	302	311	320	328	337	346	355
80	164	173	182	191	200	209	218	228	237	246	255	264	273	282	291	300	309	319	328	337	346	355	364
81	168	177	187	196	205	215	224	233	243	252	261	271	280	289	299	308	317	327	336	345	355	364	373
82	172	182	191	201	210	220	230	239	249	258	268	277	287	296	306	316	325	335	344	354	363	373	383

Code: BMI under 19: Underweight   BMI 19–24: Healthy weight   BMI 25–29 Overweight
BMI 30–39: Obesity   BMI 40 and above: Extreme obesity

Calcium-Rich, Potassium-Rich, and Magnesium-Rich Foods

Calcium-Rich Foods
Dairy: cheese, cottage cheese, milk, yogurt
Vegetables: bok choi, broccoli, kale
Beans: soybeans, tofu
Seafood: sardines and other fish with bones

Potassium-Rich Foods

Vegetables: artichoke, asparagus, avocado, bamboo shoot, beans, beet, broccoli, Brussels sprouts, carrot, cauliflower, celery, kale, mushroom, okra, potato, pumpkin, seaweed, spinach, squash (winter), sweet potato, tomato, turnip greens

Fruits: apple, apricot, avocado, banana, cantaloupe, date, dried fruit, grapefruit, honeydew, kiwifruit, orange, peach, pear, prune, strawberry, tangerine

Nuts: almonds, Brazil nuts, cashews, chestnuts, filberts, hazelnuts, peanuts, pecans, pumpkin seeds, sunflower seeds, walnuts

Cereals and breads: bran cereals, Mueslix, pumpernickel bread

Meat and poultry: pork and, at lower amounts, beef, poultry

Seafood: clams, cod, crab, halibut, lobster, rainbow trout, rockfish, salmon, tuna

Dairy: milk, yogurt

Miscellaneous: coffee, molasses, tea, tofu

Magnesium-Rich Foods

Fruits and vegetables: avocado, banana, beans, beet greens, black-eyed peas, cassava, fig, lentils, okra, potato with skin, raisins, seaweed, spinach, Swiss chard, wax beans

Whole grains: amaranth, barley, bran, brown rice, buckwheat, bulgur, granola, millet, oats, rye, triticale, whole wheat, wild rice

Dairy: milk, yogurt

Nuts: almonds, Brazil nuts, cashews, flaxseeds, hazel nuts, macadamia nuts, peanuts, pecans, pistachios, pumpkin seeds, sesame seeds, soybeans, sunflower seeds, walnuts

Seafood: cod, halibut, lobster, salmon, tuna

Food Serving Tracker

Serving Sizes and Daily Targets	Monday	Tuesday	Wednesday	Thursday	Friday	Saturday	Sunday
Vegetables: ½ cup cooked veggies, 1 cup leafy greens and raw veggies, ½ cup vegetable juice **Target:** At least 4–5 servings	☐☐☐☐☐☐	☐☐☐☐☐☐	☐☐☐☐☐☐	☐☐☐☐☐☐	☐☐☐☐☐☐	☐☐☐☐☐☐	☐☐☐☐☐☐
Fruits: ½ cup juice, small fruit, ¼ cup dried fruit, 1 cup diced raw fruit, 4 ounces raw fruit, ½ cup canned fruit **Target:** 3–5 servings	☐☐☐☐☐	☐☐☐☐☐	☐☐☐☐☐	☐☐☐☐☐	☐☐☐☐☐	☐☐☐☐☐	☐☐☐☐☐
Dairy (low-fat or nonfat): 1 cup milk, 6–8 ounces yogurt, 1 ounce cheese, ½ cup cottage cheese **Target:** At least 2–3 servings	☐☐☐☐	☐☐☐☐	☐☐☐☐	☐☐☐☐	☐☐☐☐	☐☐☐☐	☐☐☐☐
Nuts, seeds: ¼ cup or 1 ounce nuts, seeds, 2 tablespoons peanut butter **Target:** At least 1 serving	☐☐☐	☐☐☐	☐☐☐	☐☐☐	☐☐☐	☐☐☐	☐☐☐
Protein: Lean meat, fish, poultry, eggs, soy meat substitutes Each ☐ equals 1 ounce, cooked 1 egg or 2 egg whites = 1 ounce **Target:** At least 5 ounces **Vegetarian target:** 1–3 ounces	☐☐☐☐☐☐☐☐☐	☐☐☐☐☐☐☐☐☐	☐☐☐☐☐☐☐☐☐	☐☐☐☐☐☐☐☐☐	☐☐☐☐☐☐☐☐☐	☐☐☐☐☐☐☐☐☐	☐☐☐☐☐☐☐☐☐
Beans: ½ cup beans (has protein of 1 ounce meat, calories of 3 ounces) **Target:** Optional **Vegetarian target:** 1–3 servings	☐☐☐	☐☐☐	☐☐☐	☐☐☐	☐☐☐	☐☐☐	☐☐☐
Grains, starches: 1 slice bread; ⅓ cup cooked pasta, rice; ½ cup cooked cereal, corn, potatoes; 1 ounce dry cereal; ½ English muffin, bun; ¼ bagel; 2 cups popcorn **Target:** 3 or more whole grain servings	☐☐☐☐☐☐	☐☐☐☐☐☐	☐☐☐☐☐☐	☐☐☐☐☐☐	☐☐☐☐☐☐	☐☐☐☐☐☐	☐☐☐☐☐☐
Fats: 1 teaspoon oil, 1 tablespoon salad dressing, ⅛ avocado **Target:** 2–3 servings	☐☐☐	☐☐☐	☐☐☐	☐☐☐	☐☐☐	☐☐☐	☐☐☐
Alcohol: 3½ ounces wine (75 cal), 12 ounces beer (150 cal), 1 shot distilled spirits (105 cal) **Target:** None. Maximum of 2 servings	☐☐	☐☐	☐☐	☐☐	☐☐	☐☐	☐☐

Tips: Count starchy veggies as both a starch and a vegetable. A 3½ ounce serving of wine can be counted as 1 fruit.

REFERENCES

Chapter 1: You Are As Young As You Eat

Cevenini, E., et al. Inflamm-ageing. *Current Opinion in Clinical Nutrition and Metabolic Care* 16, no. 1 (2013): 14–20.

Danby, F. W. Nutrition and aging skin: sugar and glycation. *Clinical Dermatology* 28 (2010): 409–411.

Editor. Eat your way to healthier, younger-looking skin: a diet rich in vitamin C and linoleic acid. *Food & Fitness Advisor* (January 2008).

Esposito, K., et al. Dietary factors, Mediterranean diet and erectile dysfunction. *Journal of Sexual Medicine* 7 (2010): 2338–2345.

Jeanmaire, C., et al. Glycation during human dermal intrinsic and actinic ageing: an in vivo and in vitro model study. *British Journal of Dermatology* 145 (2001): 10–18.

Chapter 2: Pump Up Plant-Based Eating

The Alpha-Tocopherol Beta Carotene Cancer Prevention Study Group. The effect of vitamin E and beta carotene on the incidence of lung cancer and other cancers in male smokers. *New England Journal of Medicine* 330, no. 15 (1994): 1029–1035.

Cherniack, E. P., et al. The potential influence of plant polyphenols on the aging process. *Forschende Komplementärmedizin* 17 (2010): 181–187.

Chondrogianni, N., et al. Anti-ageing and rejuvenating effects of quercetin. *Experimental Gerontology* 45 (2010): 763–771.

Cosgrove, M. C., et al. Dietary nutrient intakes and skin-aging appearance among middle-aged American women. *American Journal of Clinical Nutrition* 86 (2007): 1225–1231.

Das, D. K., et al. Resveratrol and red wine, healthy heart and longevity. *Heart Failure Reviews* 15 (2010): 467–477.

Harman, D. Free radical theory of aging: an update: increasing the functional life span. *Annals of the New York Academy of Sciences* 1067 (2006): 10–21.

Moyer, V. A. Vitamin, mineral, and multivitamin supplementation for the primary prevention of cardiovascular disease and cancer: U.S. Preventive Services Task Force Recommendation Statement. *Annals of Internal Medicine* (February 25, 2014).

Orlich, M. J., et al. Vegetarian dietary patterns and mortality in Adventist Health Study 2. *JAMA Internal Medicine* 173 (2013): 1230–1238.

Ornish, D., et al. Effect of comprehensive lifestyle changes on telomerase activity and telomere length in men with biopsy-proven low-risk prostate cancer: 5-year follow-up of a descriptive pilot study. *Lancet Oncology* 14 (2013): 1112–1120.

Rolls, BJ, et al. Energy density but not fat content of foods affected energy intake in lean and obese women. *American Journal of Clinical Nutrition* 69, no. 5 (1999): 863–871.

Chapter 3: Brighten Your Plate with the Colors of Youth

Cox, D. C. Thirty power foods: these foods can help you slow aging, prevent disease, and boost immunity. *Natural Health* (March 2003).

Del Rio, D., G. Borges, and A. Crozier. Berry flavonoids and phenolics: bioavailability and evidence of protective effects. *British Journal of Nutrition* 104 (October 2010): S67–S90.

Proteggente, A. R., et al. The antioxidant activity of regularly consumed fruit and vegetables reflects their phenolic and vitamin C composition. *Free Radical Research* 36 (2002): 217–233.

Sadakata, S., et al. Mortality among female practitioners of Chanyou (Japanese "tea-ceremony"). *Tohoku Journal of Experimental Medicine* 166 (1992): 475–477.

Sheu, J. R., et al. Mechanisms involved in the antiplatelet activity of rutin, a glycoside of the flavonol quercetin, in human platelets. *Journal of Agricultural Food Chemistry* 52 (2004): 4414–4418.

Valdes, A. M., et al. Obesity, cigarette smoking, and telomere length in women. *Lancet* 366 (2005): 662–664.

Chapter 4: Detox with a Healthy Microbiota

Biagi, E., et al. Ageing and gut microbes: perspectives for health maintenance and longevity. *Pharmacology Research* 69 (2013): 11–20.

Claesson, M. J., et al. Gut microbiota composition correlates with diet and health in the elderly. *Nature* 488 (2012): 178–184.

Gueniche, A., et al. Probiotics for photoprotection. *Dermatoendocrinology* 1 (2009): 275–279.

Mackowiak, P. A. Recycling Metchnikoff: Probiotics, the intestinal microbiome and the Quest for Long Life. *Frontiers in Public Health* 1 (2013): 52.

Woodmansey, E. J. Intestinal bacteria and ageing. *Journal of Applied Microbiology* 102 (2007): 1178–1186.

Chapter 5: Kick Out Bad Sugars

American Heart Association. Combo of overweight, high sodium intake speeds cell aging in teens. blog.heart.org (March 20, 2014).

Gaby, A. R. Adverse effects of dietary fructose. *Alternative Medicine Review* 10 (2005): 294–306.

Hofmann, S. M., and M. H. Tschop. Dietary sugars: a fat difference. *Journal of Clinical Investigation* 119 (2009): 1089–1092.

Liu, H., and A. P. Heaney. Refined fructose and cancer. *Expert Opinion on Therapeutic Targets* 15 (2011): 1049–1059.

Marriott, B. P., N. Cole, and E. Lee. National estimates of dietary fructose intake increased from 1977 to 2004 in the United States. *The Journal of Nutrition* (June 2009): 1228S-1235S.

Sansom, W. New analysis suggests "diet soda paradox"—less sugar, more weight. UT Health Science Center, San Antonio press release, vol. 37, issue 2 (June 14, 2005).

Chapter 6: Fire Big Food and Big Pharma

Editor. Dietary supplementation with n-3 polyunsaturated fatty acids and vitamin E after myocardial infarction: results of the GISSI-Prevenzione trial. Gruppo Italiano per lo Studio della Sopravvivenza nell'Infarto miocardico. *Lancet* 354 (1999): 447–455.

Nettleton, J. A., et al. Dietary patterns, food groups, and telomere length in the Multi-Ethnic Study of Atherosclerosis (MESA). *American Journal of Clinical Nutrition* 88 (2008): 1405–1412.

Payton, S. Prostate cancer: new data risks of selenium and vitamin E. *Nature Reviews. Urology* (March 11, 2014).

Chapter 9: Three Lifestyle Secrets to a Younger You

Cherkas, L. F., et al. The association between physical activity in leisure time and leukocyte telomere length. *Archives of Internal Medicine* 168 (2008): 154–158.

Cribbett, M. R., et al. Cellular aging and restorative processes: subjective sleep quality and duration moderate the association between age and telomere length in a sample of middle-aged and older adults. *SLEEP* 37 (2014): 65–70.

Fitarone, M. A., et al. High-intensity strength training in nonagenarians. Effects on skeletal muscle. *JAMA* 263 (1990): 3029–3034.

Hoge, E. A., et al. Loving-Kindness Meditation practice associated with longer telomeres in women. *Brain, Behavior, and Immunity* 32 (2013): 159–163.

Kadi, F., et al. The effects of regular strength training on telomere length in human skeletal muscle. *Medicine & Science in Sports & Exercise* 40 (2008): 82–87.

Knutson, K. L., et al. The Metabolic Consequences of Sleep Deprivation. *Sleep Medicine Reviews* 11, no. 3 (2007): 163–178.

Okereke, O. I., et al. High phobic anxiety is related to lower leukocyte telomere length in women. *PLOS ONE* (July 11, 2012).

Ornish, D., et al. Effect of comprehensive lifestyle changes on telomerase activity and telomere length in men with biopsy-proven low-risk prostate cancer: 5-year follow-up of a descriptive pilot study. *Lancet Oncology* 14 (2013): 1112–1120.

Tuomilehto, H., et al. Sleep-disordered breathing is related to an increased risk for type 2 diabetes in middle-aged men, but not in women—the FIN-D2D survey. *Diabetes, Obesity & Metabolism* 10 (2008): 468–475.

Chapter 10: Stop the Diseases of Aging

Chiu, K. C., et al. Hypovitaminosis D is associated with insulin resistance and beta cell dysfunction. *American Journal of Clinical Nutrition* 79 (2004): 820–825.

Debette, S., et al. Midlife vascular risk factor exposure accelerates structural brain aging and cognitive decline. *Neurology* 77 (2011): 461–468.

Editor. 9 drug types that may hurt your sex life: knowing which medications may cause sexual side effects. *Men's Health Advisor* (November 2007).

Galli, R. L., et al. Fruit polyphenolics and brain aging: nutritional interventions targeting age-related neuronal and behavioral deficits. *Annals of the New York Academy of Sciences* 959 (2002): 128–132.

Hilpert, K. F., et al. Effects of dairy products on intracellular calcium and blood pressure in adults with essential hypertension. *Journal of the American College of Nutrition* 28 (2009): 142–149.

Keli, S. O., et al. Dietary flavonoids, antioxidant vitamins, and incidence of stroke: the Zutphen study. *Archives of Internal Medicine* 156 (1996): 637–642.

Nicholson, A. S., et al. Toward improved management of NIDDM: A randomized, controlled, pilot intervention using a lowfat, vegetarian diet. *Preventive Medicine* 29 (1999): 87–91.

Pankow, J. S. Metabolic syndrome risk for cardiovascular disease and diabetes in the ARIC study. *International Journal of Obesity* (May 2008).

Smith, P. J., et al. Effects of the dietary approaches to stop hypertension diet, exercise, and caloric restriction on neurocognition in overweight adults with high blood pressure. *Hypertension* 55 (2010): 1331–1338.

Wengreen, H., et al. Prospective study of Dietary Approaches to Stop Hypertension– and Mediterranean-style dietary patterns and age-related cognitive change: the Cache County Study on Memory, Health and Aging. *American Journal of Clinical Nutrition* 98 (2013): 1263–1271.

INDEX

ABOUT THE AUTHOR

MARLA HELLER, MS, RD, is a registered dietitian and holds a master of science in human nutrition and dietetics from the University of Illinois at Chicago (UIC), where she also completed doctoral course work in public health. Marla worked as a dietitian at the University of Illinois Medical Center in the Heart-Lung Transplant Unit, the Cardiac Intensive Care Unit, and the Cardiac Step-Down Unit. She has taught nutrition courses at UIC and Dominican University, and taught nutrition to student chefs at the Cooking and Hospitality Institute of Chicago. She was a civilian dietitian with the U.S. Navy and worked for the U.S. Department of Health and Human Services.

In addition to writing the *New York Times* bestsellers *The DASH Diet Action Plan, The DASH Diet Weight Loss Solution,* and *The Everyday DASH Diet Cookbook,* Marla contributed the four-week menu plan for *Win the Weight Game* by Sarah, the Duchess of York. Marla has been a featured nutrition expert for many national print, television, radio, Internet, and social media platforms, including her own PBS special on the DASH diet. She has been a spokesperson for the Greater Midwest Affiliate of the American Heart Association and a past president of the Illinois Dietetic Association.

Marla lives with her husband, Richard, and enjoys cooking, gardening, and finding exciting new restaurants.